Intercollegiate MRCS
An Aid to the VIVA
Examination

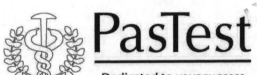

PasTest

Dedicated to your success

Intercollegiate MRCS
An Aid to the VIVA
Examination

Manoj Ramachandran
BSc(Hons) MBBS(Hons) MRCS(Eng)
FRCS(Tr&Orth)
Specialist Orthopaedic Registrar
Royal National Orthopaedic Hospital
London

Alex Malone
BSc(Hons) MBBS MRCS(Eng)
FRCS(Tr&Orth)
Specialist Orthopaedic Registrar
Royal National Orthopaedic Hospital
London

Christopher Chan
BSc(Hons) MBBS FRCS
Consultant Colorectal and General Surgeon
Barts and The London NHS Trust
London

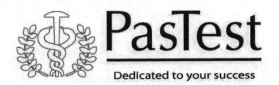

PasTest

Dedicated to your success

First published 2005

ISBN: 1904 627 498

A catalogue record for this book is available from the British Library.

The information contained within this book was obtained by the author from reliable sources. However, while every effort has been make to ensure its accuracy, no responsibility for loss, damage or injury occasioned to any person acting or refraining from action as a result of information contained herein can be accepted by the publishers or author.

PasTest Revision Books and Intensive Courses

PasTest has been established in the field of postgraduate medical education since 1972, providing revision books and intensive study courses for doctors preparing for their professional examinations.

Books and courses are available for the following specialties:

MRCGP, MRCP Parts 1 and 2, MRCPCH Parts 1 and 2, MRCPsych, MRCS, MRCOG Parts 1 and 2, DRCOG, DCH, FRCA, PLAB Parts 1 and 2.

For further details contact:

PasTest, Freepost, Knutsford, Cheshire WA16 7BR
Tel: 01565 752000   Fax: 01565 650264
www.pastest.co.uk   enquiries@pastest.co.uk

Text prepared by Type Study, Scarborough, North Yorkshire
Printed and bound in the UK by MPG Books, Cornwall

Contents

Contents

Foreword

The MRCS examination has evolved considerably since its original introduction, based on best practice, with regard to the objective assessment of medical education. The recent introduction of an Intercollegiate examination is a welcome and long overdue development. The chronology of the viva and clinical sections of the examination has been changed. This change emphasises the 'gatekeeper' role of the viva and the singular importance of the clinical section.

Many 'Aids' have been published to facilitate the examination process with variable success. The PasTest series, established for over 30 years, has an excellent pedigree. The particular attributes of this book include the care taken to ensure the topics detailed reflect those commonly encountered in the examination and the use of structured topic developments from basic through to advanced knowledge.

The authors have extensive experience in publishing examination companion texts as well as an infectious enthusiasm for 'hands on' teaching courses, which I have witnessed first hand. Their expertise and enthusiasm is evident in this book, which will prove highly useful for surgical trainees and budding undergraduates alike.

Professor Marc Winslet MS FRCS
Professor of Surgery, Head of Department and Chairman of Division of Surgery and Interventional Sciences, Royal Free & University College Medical School, University College London

About the authors

Manoj Ramachandran is a Specialist Orthopaedic Registrar based at the Royal National Orthopaedic Hospital in Stanmore. He qualified from King's College Hospital Medical School, London with multiple honours in 1996 and was *proxime accessit* to the University of London Gold Medal. He completed his basic surgical training on the Oxford and Hammersmith rotations, and became a Member of the Royal College of Surgeons of England in 1999 and a Fellow (Trauma and Orthopaedics) in 2005. He is the author of a successful clinical book entitled *Clinical Cases and OSCEs in Surgery* and has been running a portfolio of surgical and career development courses since 1999, which he plans to continue in his capacity as Honorary Lecturer at the Royal Free Medical School with the Department of Surgery.

Alex Malone is a Specialist Orthopaedic Registrar based at the Royal National Orthopaedic Hospital in Stanmore. He qualified from St Mary's Medical School, London in 1996, completed basic surgical training and became a Member of the Royal College of Surgeons of England in 1999 and a Fellow (Trauma and Orthopaedics) in 2005. He has taught, designed and directed MRCS courses since 2001 and has recently been appointed as Honorary Lecturer at the Royal Free Medical School, to set up a portfolio of medical education courses with the Department of Surgery.

Christopher Chan is a Consultant Colorectal and General Surgeon based at Barts and The London NHS Trust. He qualified from the United Medical and Dental Schools of Guys and St Thomas', having completed his general surgical training in Cambridge and London and his specialist colorectal training in London and Sydney, Australia. He is an invited lecturer at the Royal College of Surgeons of England and Final FRCS Fellowship courses. He has taught on MRCS courses since 1997 and was MRCS Course Director from 2000–2002. He has contributed as an author to a number of successful MRCS publications, including Intercollegiate *MRCS: Applied Basic Science MCQs; Intercollegiate MRCS: Clinical Problem-Solving Volume 1;* and *VIVA Practice for Intercollegiate MRCS (Part 3).*

Acknowledgements

This book is dedicated to all the tutors and contributors who have taught on MRCS Viva courses organised by Manoj Ramachandran and Alex Malone, without whom this would have been impossible to put together. This book is as much theirs as it is ours.

We would also like to thank Kirsten Baxter and Amy Smith for their hard work, speed and efficiency. They are a credit to PastTest and contributory to its continuing success.

Contributors

Rachel Bell
John Bycroft
Ramesh Chelvarajah
Alex Cheung
Kenan Deniz
Rupinder Deol
Deborah Eastwood
Callum Faris
Victoria Giblin
Alister Hart
John Hewitt
Tariq Hoth
Azhar Khan
Kelvin Lau
Joshua Lee
Kathryn McCarthy
Adam Poole
Tom Quick
Kanthan Theivendran
Aaron Trinidade

Introduction

The MRCS exam is at present the major hurdle between Basic Surgical Training and progression to Higher Surgical Training (or, in the near future, progression within a foundation programme structure). Until recently, the clinical component of the MRCS was the first step in passing the second and final part of the exam, but this has been changed recently and candidates now have to pass the viva before they are allowed to progress to the final clinical examination. The viva is regarded as the toughest component of the MRCS exam. Previously, there were two sittings per year for each of the individual Royal Colleges (London, Edinburgh, Glasgow and Dublin) for the MRCS viva, but now the intercollegiate MRCS exam has three sittings per year, with plans to increase the number at overseas centres.

The contents of this book are based on the structure of the MRCS viva itself, with every question having been carefully vetted and accurately researched before inclusion. The topics closely reflect those in the MRCS viva itself. Within each section, there are approximately 30 questions with answers in bullet form, except for the communication skills section, where there are ten scenarios with model answers.

Each question has three levels (an entry question, a development question and an advanced question), usually progressing in difficulty with each question. We hope that the reader uses the questions as a base to build knowledge on and to practice the necessary techniques for the viva voce examination.

The unique features of this book include:

- It is relevant to the new exam (including intercollegiate changes).
- It is written in a format that closely resembles the exam.
- It covers most common topics.

This book is primarily aimed at those doctors who are in Basic Surgical Training or who are newly appointed Foundation-Year trainees who are sitting the viva component of the MRCS exam. The book will also be of great value to medical students preparing for undergraduate finals and to Specialist Registrars in all surgical specialties preparing for their exit examinations.

1

CLINICAL PATHOLOGY

1   ACUTE INFLAMMATION

What are the features of acute inflammation?

The five cardinal features of acute inflammation are:

1   Rubor (redness)
2   Calor (heat)
3   Dolor (pain)
4   Tumor (swelling)
5   Functio laesa (loss of function).

What is the sequence of events that takes place in acute inflammation?

The initial phase is vasoconstriction, followed immediately by vasodilatation with increased vascular permeability.

Further events include:

- Leucocytic margination and emigration (neutrophils first and then monocytes)
- Phagocytosis, involving:
  - intracellular degradation of ingested particles (oxygen-dependent and oxygen-independent)
  - extracellular release of leucocyte products, eg lysosomal enzymes.

What are the outcomes of acute inflammation?

The three most common outcomes are:

- Complete resolution
- Healing by scarring
- Progression to chronic inflammation.

2   CHRONIC INFLAMMATION

Chronic inflammation may have a variety of causes. Can you name some?

Common causes of chronic inflammation include:

- Persistent infection by intracellular microbes (eg tubercle bacilli), which are of low toxicity but evoke an immunological reaction
- Prolonged exposure to non-degradable but potentially toxic substances, eg silica, asbestos
- Autoimmune reactions.

What are the key cells in chronic inflammation?

- Mononuclear cells, principally macrophages and lymphocytes
- Eosinophils (in immune reactions).

How do macrophages and lymphocytes interact in chronic inflammation?

Macrophages are the principal cells involved in chronic inflammation. They are activated by lymphokines (eg γ interferon) produced by immune activated T cells or by immune factors, such as exotoxin. The secretory products of macrophages induce characteristic chronic inflammatory changes, including:

- Tissue destruction (proteases and oxygen-derived free radicals)
- Neovascularisation
- Fibroblast proliferation
- Connective tissue growth (IL-1, TNF-α).

Lymphocytes have a reciprocal relationship with macrophages in chronic inflammation. Activated lymphocytes produce lymphokines, and these (particularly γ interferon) are the major stimulators of macrophages. Activated macrophages produce monokines, which in turn influence B- and T-helper cell function.

3   NECROSIS

What is necrosis?

Definition: Necrosis is abnormal tissue death and is the sum of the morphological changes that follow cell death in living tissue or organs. It is energy-independent and stimulates an inflammatory response (**unlike apoptosis, which is programmed cell death**).

The pathological processes involved in necrosis are:

- Denaturation of proteins
- Enzymatic digestion of organelles and cytosol, either through autolysis (by lysosomes of dead cells themselves) or by heterolysis (digestion by lysosomes of immigrant leucocytes).

What different types of necrosis do you know of?

The pattern of necrosis is dependent on the balance of denaturation and digestion:

Coagulation/structured necrosis: more denaturation of proteins than digestion, so the tissue architecture is preserved. Seen in kidney, myocardium, liver and spleen.

Colliquative/liquefactive necrosis: autolysis and heterolysis of proteins prevail over denaturation of proteins. Tends to occur in tissues rich in lipid where lysosomal enzymes denature fat and cause liquefaction, for example the brain and localised bacterial infections (abscesses).

Caseous/unstructured necrosis: gross appearance is of soft, cheesy, friable material and microscopically appears as amorphous debris. Tissue architecture is lost. Coagulated proteins and degenerate lipid components are seen. Classically seen in tuberculosis.

Fat necrosis: induced by the action of lipases that catalyse decomposition of triglycerides to fatty acids, which then complex with calcium to create calcium soaps. Seen following breast trauma and pancreatitis.

Gangrene is also a form of necrosis and can be either:

- **Wet gangrene** (putrefaction due to anaerobic bacteria such as *Bacteroides* or *Clostridium* species), or
- **Dry gangrene** (mummification of a tissue without infection, eg toes in a diabetic patient).

What cellular changes are seen during necrosis?

- The necrotic cell becomes eosinophilic and glassy and vacuolation may be seen.
- Cell membrane fragmentation.
- Nuclear changes, including:
  - pyknosis (small, dense nucleus)
  - karyolysis (faint, dissolved nucleus)
  - karyorrhexis (nucleus broken up into many clumps).
- Mitochondria are swollen and large, with amorphous densities.
- Rupture of lysosomes.
- Rupture of endoplasmic reticulum.

Note that in **reversible cell injury**, clumping of nuclear chromatin is seen, along with detachment of ribosomes from the endoplasmic reticulum, and formation of membrane blebs and myelin figures, which can all be reversed if oxygenation is restored.

4   CALCIFICATION

What different types of calcification exist?

- **Orthotopic:** a normal process in bone, teeth and otoliths
- **Heterotopic:**
  - dystrophic
  - metastatic
  - age-related (this is dystrophic in some cases).

What is the difference between dystrophic and metastatic calcification?

Dystrophic calcification is seen in non-viable or dying tissues in the presence of normal serum calcium levels.

Metastatic calcification is seen in vital tissues where deposition of calcium salts occurs in association with hypercalcaemia.

Can you give some examples of dystrophic and metastatic calcification?

Dystrophic calcification: most commonly seen in damaged heart valves, damaged muscle, atheroma, scars, in areas of necrosis (coagulative, caseous and liquefactive) and parasitic cysts (eg cysticercosis). Calcium deposition can be intracellular, extracellular or both.

Two phases are seen:

- **Initiation phase**, which occurs extracellularly due to membrane-bound vesicles concentrating calcium or intracellularly within mitochondria
- **Propagation phase**, where crystal formation occurs, depending on the concentration of calcium and phosphates, the presence of mineral inhibitors, and the presence of collagen.

Metastatic calcification: tends to occur in areas where acidic substances are excreted. Common areas include: around the gastric glands (where hydrochloric acid is secreted), the renal tubules, ie nephrocalcinosis (where hydrogen ions are secreted), and the lung (where carbon dioxide is secreted). Hypercalcaemia itself may give rise to metastatic calcification, as in hyperparathyroidism, metastatic carcinomas and systemic sarcoidosis.

5   ATROPHY, HYPERTROPHY AND HYPERPLASIA

What do you understand by the term 'atrophy' and what causes it?

Definition: Atrophy is the shrinkage in the size of cells and tissues due to loss of cell substance. The cells have diminished function but are not dead.

Cells exhibit autophagy, with a reduction in the number of cell organelles, and a marked increase in the number of autophagic vacuoles. Components that resist digestion are converted to lipofuscin granules that, in sufficient numbers, make the organ brown ('brown atrophy').

Causes of atrophy include normal ageing, decreased workload, loss of innervation, reduced blood supply, diminished nutrition and loss of endocrine stimulation.

What do you understand by the term 'hypertrophy' and can you give some examples?

Definition: Hypertrophy is an increase in the number of organelles and the **size of cells** and, as a result of such changes, an increase in the size of the organ.

Hypertrophy can be **physiological** or **pathological**.

Causes of hypertrophy include:

- Increased functional demand, eg hypertrophy of skeletal muscles with exercise (physiological) or of muscle in disease, eg cardiomyopathy and congenital muscular dystrophies (both pathological)
- Specific hormonal stimulation eg uterine hypertrophy in pregnancy (physiological) or Graves' disease (pathological).

What do you understand by the term 'hyperplasia' and can you give some examples?

Definition: Hyperplasia is an increase in the **number of cells** in an organ or tissue. It may be accompanied by hypertrophy, as in prostatic and adrenal enlargement.

Hyperplasia only occurs in cells that are capable of synthesising DNA. Nerve, cardiac and skeletal muscle cells can undergo almost pure hypertrophy when stimulated by hormones or by increased functional demand.

Hyperplasia may be **physiological** or **pathological**:

- **Physiological hyperplasia** can be either **hormonal** (eg breast, thyroid and pituitary in pregnancy and endometrial hyperplasia after oestrogen stimulation) or **compensatory** (eg hyperplasia of the liver after partial hepatectomy).

- **Pathological hyperplasia** can be either **hormonal** (eg atypical endometrial hyperplasia seen with excessive oestrogen) or secondary to locally produced **growth factors** (eg squamous epithelium induced by human papillomavirus).

6   ABSCESS

What is an abscess?

Definition: An abscess is a loculated or localised collection of pus lined by granulation tissue.

What are the constituents of pus?

Pus has solid and fluid phases:

- The **solid phase** contains live and dead polymorphs, occasionally macrophages, live and dead bacteria, dead human cells from the involved tissues and fibrin meshwork.
- The **fluid phase** consists of exudates and carries immunoglobulins, complement components, clotting cascade factors and other inflammatory mediators, including arachidonic acid, kinins and cytokines.

Sterile abscesses do not contain micro-organisms and may be seen following intramuscular injections.

What happens to abscesses if they are left untreated?

Abscesses eventually discharge through the site of least resistance. This occurs as a result of an increase in osmotic pressure within the abscess following enzyme release by polymorphs and macrophages, causing long-chain molecules to be spilt into smaller molecules. These numerous smaller molecules produce the increase in osmotic pressure.

7   ISCHAEMIA AND INFARCTION

What is the difference between ischaemia and infarction?

Ischaemia is an abnormal reduction in the blood supply to, or drainage from, an organ or tissue.

Infarction is the result of the reduction in the blood supply to, or drainage from, an organ or tissue.

Can you list some causes of ischaemia and infarction?

Generalised causes of ischaemia and infarction:

• Hypoxaemia
• Anaemia.

Localised causes of ischaemia and infarction:

• Arterial obstruction, eg thrombus, embolus, vasospasm and external compression, as with tourniquet use
• Venous obstruction, eg thrombus, stasis, pressure sores or intussusception
• Capillary obstruction, eg vasculitis in meningococcal septicaemia
• Miscellaneous, eg sickle cell disease, malaria, fat embolism, caisson disease, frostbite.

With respect to arterial causes, what factors increase the severity of the infarction?

• Tissue involved, eg brain and heart are more vulnerable than skeletal muscle and skin
• Speed of onset
• Degree of obstruction/stenosis of lumen
• Presence of collateral blood supply
• Level of oxygenation of the blood
• Systemic disorders, eg heart failure
• Microvascular disease, eg diabetes mellitus.

8   WOUND HEALING

What are the phases of wound healing?

Coagulative and substrate phase:

- Fibrin clot (acting as a matrix) fills the wound, and platelets degranulate, releasing transforming growth factor β (TGF-β) and platelet derived growth factor (PDGF).

Inflammatory phase:

- Neutrophils enter the wound matrix and phagocytose contaminating bacteria and debris. This is followed by vessel contraction and platelet plugging.

Synthesis phase:

- Migration of monocytes as a result of chemotaxis. Monocytes differentiate into macrophages that further phagocytose debris and produce more growth factors.

Remodelling phase:

- Fibroblasts migrate into the wound and produce collagen and glycoproteins for the extracellular matrix.
- Angiogenesis occurs, resulting in the formation of granulation tissue.

Maturation phase:

- Myofibroblasts contract the wound.
- Scar tissue forms due to continuous collagen deposition and degradation by matrix proteinases.

Epithelialisation phase:

- Keratinocytes migrate through and attach to the wound matrix, as well as dividing and encroaching from the wound edge, controlled by basic fibroblast growth factor (FGF) and epidermal growth factor (EGF).

What is the difference between healing by primary intention and healing by secondary intention?

Primary intention: There is no tissue loss and the wound is often closed by means of sutures. This may be by:

- Primary closure (closed at time of trauma or surgery), or
- Delayed primary closure (3–4 days later when the wound is free of potentially infecting organisms).

Secondary intention: This occurs in wounds with tissue loss. Healing is via the formation of granulation tissue that fills the area of tissue loss.

What is the difference between hypertrophic and keloid scars?

	Hypertrophic scars	Keloid scars
Appearance	Scar confined to wound margins	Scar extends beyond wound margins
Site	Across flexor surfaces and skin creases	Ear lobes, chin, neck, shoulder, chest
Age group	Any age (commonly 8–20 years)	Puberty to 30 years
Gender	M = F	F > M
Racial groups affected	All races	Black and Hispanic races
Biochemical features	Normal rate of collagen synthesis but increased breakdown of collagen by collagenase activity	Increased rate of collagen synthesis (increased proline hydroxylase activity); increased collagenase activity
Genetic links	Not proven	Significant predisposition in Black and Hispanic races
Oxygen levels	Relative hypoxia, possibly due to wound tension	No link
Immunology	May be important, but no specific associations known	Increased IgG, IgM and C3 levels; antinuclear antibodies to keloid fibroblasts

9 GRANULOMATOUS INFLAMMATION

What is a granuloma?

Definition: A collection of modified macrophages surrounded by a rim of lymphocytes, often with multinucleated giant cells. When epithelioid cells (modified macrophages) coalesce, they form multinucleate giant cells.

Can you name any granulomatous diseases?

- Bacterial, eg tuberculosis, leprosy, syphilis, cat-scratch disease
- Parasitic, eg schistosomiasis
- Fungal, eg *Cryptococcus neoformans*
- Inorganic metals and dusts, eg silicosis, berylliosis
- Unknown, eg sarcoidosis.

What types of giant cells do you know?

Normal giant cells:

- Osteoclasts
- Skeletal muscle cells
- Megakaryocytes
- Syncytiotrophoblasts.

Abnormal giant cells:

- Macrophage-related, eg Langhans' cells in tuberculosis, sarcoidosis and Crohn's disease
- Virus-induced, eg herpes simplex
- Tumour-related, eg Reed–Sternberg cells in Hodgkin's disease
- Miscellaneous, eg megaloblasts in folate and vitamin B_{12} deficiency.

10   TUMOUR MARKERS

What is a tumour marker?

Definition: A tumour marker is a substance produced by a tumour that is present in the blood or other tissues. It may be useful in:

- Aiding in diagnosis
- Monitoring the response to treatment
- Indicating recurrence
- Aiding in prognosis.

What types of tumour markers do you know?

Many chemical groups are represented, examples of which are:

- **Hormones** – cortisol, adrenocorticotrophic hormone (ACTH)
- **Antigens** – carcinoembryonic antigen (CEA, an oncofetal antigen), α-fetoprotein
- **Amino and nucleic acids** – vanillylmandelic acid (VMA), 5-hydroxyindoleacetic acid (5-HIAA)
- **Enzymes:** prostate-specific antigen (PSA), prostate acid phosphatase
- **Polyamines** – calcitonin
- **Specific cell membrane:** insulin-like growth factor 1 (IGF-1).

Can you give examples of clinically useful tumour markers?

Examples include:

- **ACTH** – ectopic hormone produced by oat-cell lung carcinoma
- **PSA** – produced by prostate tumours; aids in the diagnosis of prostate cancer
- **CEA** – used for follow-up of recurrence of colorectal carcinoma
- **α-Fetoprotein** – produced by primary liver tumours and testicular teratomas
- **VMA** – increased levels in the urine of patients with phaeochromocytoma
- **5-HIAA** – increased levels in carcinoid tumours
- **calcitonin** – aids in the diagnosis of thyroid medullary carcinoma
- **cortisol** – produced by adrenal tumours
- **IGF-1** – increased in brain tumours, especially gliomas.

11   ENDOTOXINS AND EXOTOXINS

What is an endotoxin?

Definition: Lipopolysaccharide from the cell wall of Gram-negative organisms. It is non-immunogenic and heat stable. Non-specific effects of endotoxin include:

- Cytokine formation
- Fibrin degradation
- Clotting cascade activation
- Nitric oxide formation
- Prostaglandin formation
- Complement activation.

What is an exotoxin?

Definition: Secreted protein that is immunogenic and heat labile. It is a characteristic of Gram-positive organisms. Specific effects include:

- Enzymatic action, eg *Vibrio cholerae* toxin
- Neurotoxic, eg tetanospasmin from *Clostridium tetani*, *Clostridium botulinum* toxin
- Destructive effects on the plasma membrane, eg *Staphylococcus aureus* toxin and *Clostridium perfringens* toxin.

Can you name some diseases or conditions caused by endotoxins and exotoxins?

Exotoxins:

- Cholera
- Diphtheria
- Gas gangrene, botulism and tetanus
- Food poisoning.

Endotoxins:

- Disseminated intravascular coagulation (DIC)
- Multiple-organ failure.

12   BLOOD GROUPS

What do you understand about the ABO blood group system?

- The ABO blood group system consists of three allelic genes – A, B and O.
- The A and B genes control the synthesis of enzymes that add carbohydrate residues to cell surface glycoproteins and the O gene is an amorph that does not transform the glycoprotein.
- There are six possible genotypes but only four phenotypes.
- Naturally-occurring antibodies are found in the serum of those lacking the corresponding antigen.

Phenotype	Genotype	Antigens	Antibodies	Frequency
O	OO	O	Anti-A, Anti-B	46%
A	AA or AO	A	Anti-B	42%
B	BB or BO	B	Anti-A	9%
AB	AB	AB	None	3%

What is blood grouping and ABO compatibility?

Blood group O = universal donor.
Blood group AB = universal recipient.

Blood group	Antigens	Antibodies	Can give blood to	Can receive blood from
AB	A and B	None	AB	AB, A, B, O
A	A	B	A and AB	A and O
B	B	A	B and AB	B and O
O	None	A and B	AB, A, B, O	O

In blood grouping, a patient's red cells are grouped for ABO and Rhesus antigens, and the serum is tested to confirm the patient's ABO group.

Tell me about the Rhesus (Rh) system?

- Rhesus antibodies are immune antibodies, requiring exposure during transfusion or pregnancy – 85% of the population is Rh-positive.
- 90% of Rh-negative patients transfused with Rh-positive blood develop anti-D antibodies.
- The two common alleles are D and d. If an individual (diploid) has both D alleles (homozygous) or just one D allele (heterozygous), they synthesise a glycolipid antigen (the Rhesus D antigen) on the surface of their red cells.
- Unlike the ABO antibodies (anti-A and anti-B), the antibody that recognises the D antigen (anti-D) is not

naturally occurring. It only arises as a result of the immunisation of a Rh-negative person (dd) with the D antigen, usually via Rh-positive (DD or Dd) blood, most commonly via transfusion or pregnancy.

13   BLOOD TRANSFUSION

What different blood products are available to you as a surgeon?

- Whole blood
- Red blood cells – packed red cells/leucocyte-depleted/ irradiated and CMV-depleted
- White blood cells – granulocyte concentrates
- Platelets – platelet concentrates
- Plasma – human plasma – fresh frozen plasma/freeze-dried plasma/plasma protein fraction/human albumin 25%/cryoprecipitate/clotting factors – factor VIII/IX/ immunoglobulins (note that serum contains no clotting factors).

What are the complications of blood transfusion?

Early complications:

- Haemolytic reactions (immediate or delayed 5–10 days)
- Bacterial infection from contamination
- Allergic reactions to white cells or platelets
- Pyogenic reactions (non-haemolytic transfusion febrile reaction)
- Circulatory overload
- Air embolism
- Thrombophlebitis
- Citrate toxicity
- Hyperkalaemia
- Clotting abnormalities
- Transfusion-related lung injury (similar to acute respiratory distress syndrome, due to the interaction of donor antibodies with recipient white cells).

Late complications:

- Infection – cytomegalovirus, hepatitis
- Immune sensitisation
- Iron overload.

How would you deal with an anaphylactic reaction when transfusing blood?

- Stop the transfusion immediately and remove the giving set.
- Maintain airway and administer 100% oxygen.
- Administer adrenaline (epinephrine) intramuscularly (0.5 ml adrenaline injection 1 in 1000), chlorphenamine (10–20 mg) slow intravenous injection and hydrocortisone (100–300 mg) intravenously.

14   HAEMOSTASIS

What do you understand by the term 'haemostasis'?

The haemostatic response has three elements:

- Vasoconstriction
- Platelet aggregation
- Clotting cascade.

What are the mechanisms involved in platelet aggregation?

- Platelets are formed in bone marrow from megakaryocytes.
- They contain the contractile proteins, actin and myosin.
- Platelets have no nucleus but contain endoplasmic reticulum and Golgi apparatus that can produce proteins.
- Platelets contain mitochondria that can produce ATP and ADP.
- Platelets can also synthesise prostaglandins and thromboxane A_2.
- They have a half-life in the blood of 8–12 days.
- In response to tissue damage, platelets undergo a number of changes.
- Platelet aggregation can result in a 'platelet plug' that can occlude a small hole.
- Platelets adhere to damaged endothelium (via von Willebrand factor).
- Aggregating platelets release arachidonic acid, which is converted to thromboxane A_2.
- Calcium-mediated contraction of actin and myosin results in degranulation.
- ADP is released, which can induce further aggregation and release in a positive-feedback fashion.

What surgical haemostatic agents are you aware of?

Natural haemostatic agents:

- Tisseel® glue (fibrin)
- Thrombin
- Surgicel® (cellulose)
- Bone wax (beeswax).

Artificial haemostatic agents:

- QuikClot®, a chemically inert haemostatic agent that accelerates coagualation of blood by physically adsorbing liquid from blood, concentrating clotting factors
- TraumaDEX™
- Spongstan®.

15   COAGULATION

What are the pathways involved in the clotting cascade?

- The clotting cascade occurs through two semi-independent pathways:
  - the intrinsic pathway, which has all of its components within blood
  - the extrinsic pathway, which is triggered by extravascular tissue damage (exposure to a tissue factor).
- Both pathways result in activation of prothrombin (Factor IIa), with the final common pathway converting fibrinogen to fibrin monomer.
- Polymerisation of fibrin results in the formation of long fine strands held together by H-bonds which are then converted into covalent bonds with stabilisation of the fibrin polymer.
- The intrinsic pathway is relatively slow (2–6 minutes), while the extrinsic pathway is much faster (15 seconds).

Can you draw the clotting cascade?

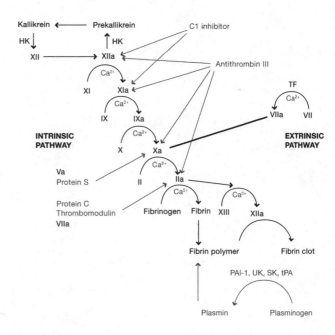

What prevents the clotting cascade from spreading uncontrollably?

- Thrombin (in the presence of fibronectin and fibrinogen) induces endothelial cell release of urokinase and tissue-type plasminogen activators (tPA) to convert plasminogen to plasmin.
- Fibrin split products formed by fibrinolysis inhibit clotting.

- Activated clotting factors are depleted by dilution at sites of clot formation.
- Activated factors are cleared by the liver and mononuclear phagocyte system.
- Thrombin unmasks endothelial cell receptors (thrombomodulin) that bind and activate protein C, which in turn inactivates Factors Va and VIIIa.

16   ANTICOAGULATION

What anticoagulants are used in daily clinical practice?

- Heparin
- Low molecular weight heparins, eg enoxaparin, dalteparin
- Warfarin
- Pentasaccharides (fondaparinux).

How does heparin work and how does this differ from the action of low molecular weight heparin (LMWH)?

Heparin (a mixture of sulphated glycosaminoglycans):

- Potentiates the action of antithrombin III, which inactivates thrombin (Factor II) and other factors (especially Xa but also XIIa and XIa) involved in the clotting cascade, which in turn inhibits thrombus formation
- Causes some inhibition of platelet function
- Increases the permeability of vessels
- Inhibits vascular smooth muscle proliferation.

LMWH:

- Acts predominantly on Factor Xa
- Does not bind to antithrombin III simultaneously, so does not inhibit thrombin as much, resulting in less bleeding
- Reduced binding to plasma cells, endothelial cells and macrophages, so increases bioavailability.

Fondaparinux has a similar action to LMWH.

How does warfarin work?

Warfarin:

- Competitively antagonises vitamin K (an essential cofactor for Factors II, VII, IX and X)
- Inhibits the synthesis of protein C and protein S
- Has no direct effect on coagulation factors already present in the blood
- In the first 24 hours causes a hypercoagulable state due to inhibition of protein C synthesis
- Has a half-life 40 hours.

17   DISSEMINATED INTRAVASCULAR COAGULATION

What do you understand by the term 'disseminated intravascular coagulation' (DIC) and what are the common causes?

Definition: DIC is the widespread intravascular activation of the clotting cascade, leading to bleeding as a result of consumption of clotting factors and activation of fibrinolytic mechanisms.

It presents with bruising, purpura or oozing from surgical wounds and venepuncture sites.

Causes of DIC:

*   Severe infection (usually Gram-negative or meningococcal)
*   Hypovolaemic shock
*   Burns
*   Transfusion reaction
*   Eclampsia
*   Amniotic fluid embolus
*   Promyelocytic leukaemia
*   Mucin-secreting metastatic adenocarcinoma.

What investigations can be used to confirm the diagnosis?

*   Increased activated partial thromboplastin time (APTT) and prothrombin time (PT)
*   Reduced serum fibrinogen levels (<1 mg/ml)
*   Thrombocytopenia
*   Increased fibrin degradation products
*   Reduced Factor V and Factor VIII activity.

How do you treat DIC?

*   Fluid resuscitation
*   Treat underlying cause
*   Correct clotting abnormalities with:
    *   fresh frozen plasma
    *   cryoprecipitate
    *   platelet transfusion.

18   SICKLE CELL ANAEMIA

What is sickle cell anaemia?

- Normal haemoglobin has two α and two β chains.
- In sickle cell disease, a single amino acid substitution occurs on the β chain (valine substituted for glutamic acid at position 6). The resulting HbS is less soluble than HbA.
- It has an autosomal recessive inheritance, affecting those of Afro-Caribbean descent.
- Sickle cell anaemia occurs in homozygotes; sickle cell trait occurs in heterozygotes.
- When deoxygenated, haemoglobin undergoes polymerisation and forms characteristic sickle cells which block small vessels, resulting in vaso-occlusive events.
- Sickling may be precipitated by infection, fever, dehydration, cold, or hypoxia.

How does sickle cell anaemia present clinically?

Sickle cell anaemia may present with acute complications, including:

- Painful crises
- Worsening anaemia (aplastic crisis with parvovirus B19 infection)
- Acute chest syndrome (*Chlamydia* and *Mycoplasma*)
- Focal neurological or ocular events
- Priapism.

Can you name some important considerations for a surgeon dealing with a sickle cell patient?

- High risk of acute sickling complications under general anaesthesia and require careful pre- and perioperative management.
- Transfusion may be required to ensure a haemoglobin of 9–10 g/dl (though preoperative exchange transfusion is rarely required).
- Tourniquets should be used with caution.
- Principles are to:
  - avoid dehydration
  - avoid hypoxia
  - control intra- and postoperative pain.

19   HYPERSPLENISM

What is hypersplenism?

Three features:

- Splenomegaly
- Reduced levels of one or more blood cell elements, resulting in anaemia, leucopenia, thrombocytopenia (or any combination thereof), in association with hyperplasia of the marrow precursors of the deficient cell type
- Correction of the cytopenia by splenectomy.

What causes of hypersplenism do you know of?

- Congestive splenomegaly, eg cirrhosis of the liver
- Infection and inflammation, eg hepatitis, sarcoidosis
- Myeloproliferative and lymphoproliferative diseases, eg lymphoma, leukaemia
- Chronic haemolytic anaemia, eg hereditary spherocytosis, thalassaemia
- Storage diseases, eg Gaucher's disease, Niemann–Pick disease
- Splenic cysts.

When is splenectomy indicated in hypersplenism?

- Haemolytic syndromes with shortened survival of abnormal red blood cells, eg hereditary spherocytosis
- Severe pancytopenia associated with massive splenomegaly, eg lipid-storage diseases
- Vascular accidents involving the spleen, eg in recurrent infections
- Mechanical encroachment on other abdominal organs
- Haemorrhagic tendency, eg hypersplenic thrombocytopenia.

20   CARCINOGENESIS

What do you understand by the term 'carcinogenesis'?

Definition: Carcinogenesis is the process that results in normal cells converting to become cells capable of forming malignant neoplasms.

What are carcinogens?

Carcinogens are agents that cause cells to transform into neoplasms when exposed to them.

What groups of carcinogens do you know of and can you give some examples?

Carcinogen group	Examples	Related cancers
Chemicals	Polycyclic hydrocarbons	Lung cancer
	Azo dyes	Bladder cancer
	Aromatic amines	Bladder cancer
Viruses	Hepatitis B, hepatitis C	Hepatocellular carcinoma
	Human papillomavirus	Cervical cancer, anal cancer
Ionizing radiation	X-rays	Skin cancer
Uranium/radon	Lung cancer	
	Radioactive iodine	Thyroid cancer
Non-ionizing radiation	Ultraviolet light	Malignant melanoma
Hormones	Anabolic steroids	Liver cancer
Toxins	Aflatoxins	Liver cancer
Parasites	Liver fluke	Cholangiocarcinoma
Industrial dusts	Asbestos	Mesothelioma

21   METASTASIS

How would you define metastasis?

Definition: The seeding of tumour cells to sites distant and detached from the original area.

What are the routes by which neoplasms metastasise?

- Lymphatics
- Bloodstream
- Trans-coelomic
- Via cerebrospinal fluid (CSF)
- Seeding during surgery.

What processes do metastases have to undergo in order to be established in recipient tissue?

- Invasion of vessel/body cavity
- Targetting of recipient organ or tissue
- Establishment of growth of metastasis within the recipient tissue by acquiring a blood supply. Factors important in establishing a blood supply include:
  - cytokine/growth factor production, eg vascular endothelial growth factor (VEGF), fibroblast growth factor (FGF), angiopoietin
  - tissue hypoxia – stimulus for angiogenesis.

22   MELANOMA

Can you name the different types of melanoma?

Superficial spreading:

- Most common.

Lentigo maligna:

- Pale brown patches with irregular outline found on hands and face (Hutchinson's melanotic freckles).

Nodular melanoma:

- Younger age group
- Deeply pigmented and may bleed or ulcerate
- Poor prognosis – invades deeply as opposed to superficially.

Acral lentiginous:

- On extremities – palms of hands/soles of feet/subungual
- Blacks and Asians.

Amelanotic:

- Rare.

How are malignant melanomas staged?

Breslow's thickness:

- <0.76 mm – low risk
- 0.76–1.5 mm – moderate risk
- >1.5 mm – high risk of metastases.

Clark's levels:

I   confined to epidermis
II   into papillary dermis
III   across papillary dermis
IV   into reticular dermis
V   into subcutaneous fat

Clinical staging:

I   no regional spread
II   satellite lesions/lymph node spread
III   distant spread

What is the embryological origin of melanomas?

- They arise from the neuroectoderm of the embryonic neural crest.
- All melanocytes have a positive dihydroxyphenylalanine (DOPA) reaction, converting DOPA into melanin, which is used as the basis for specific testing.

23   BREAST CANCER

What is the current screening policy for breast cancer in the UK?

- Mammography is offered to all women aged 50–64 years every 3 years.
- After the age of 64 years, women are asked to make their own appointments if desired.
- Plans are to increase the age group for regular screening to 70 years.

What is the epidemiology of, and risk factors associated with breast cancer?

Epidemiology:

- It is the commonest cancer amongst women in the Western world.
- There are 30,000 new cases a year in the UK.
- There are 15,000 deaths annually.
- Around 1% of breast cancers occur in men.

Risk factors:

- Increasing age
- First pregnancy >30 years.
- Non-breast feeding mothers
- Early menarche, late menopause
- Hormone replacement therapy (HRT)
- Oral contraceptive pill (OCP)
- Previous breast cancer
- *BRCA1* and *BRCA2* genes.

Why is routine breast screening only offered to patients over the age of 50?

- Mammography is unreliable at picking up cancers in the breasts of younger women due to high tissue density.
- It is more effective after breast involution, which occurs at the time of menopause.
- The average age of menopause in the UK is 50 years.

24   LUNG CANCER

Describe the epidemiology and name the risk factors associated with lung cancer.

Epidemiology:

• Approximately 19% of all cancers; 27% of all cancer deaths
• Most common primary malignant tumour in the UK
• Third of all male cancers; second commonest cancer in women
• Peak age 40–70 years.

Risk factors:

• Smoking
• Age
• Asbestos/iron/iron oxides/nickel/arsenic/chromium/coal tar
• Radiation.

How are lung cancers classified?

Lung cancers may be primary or secondary.

Primary:

• Squamous cell carcinoma:
  • strongest association with smoking
  • occurs in hilar regions
• Small (oat) cell carcinoma:
  • usually arises in the hilar region
  • metastasise early and produce large deposits
• Adenocarcinoma:
  • peripheral
  • associated with pulmonary fibrosis, honeycomb lung, asbestosis
• Large-cell carcinoma:
  • centrally placed and aggressive
  • associated necrosis and haemorrhage.

Secondary: metastases from breast, lung, sarcoma, colon, kidneys.

What are the clinical consequences of local invasion of lung cancer?

Structure invaded	Consequence
Sympathetic chain	Horner's syndrome
Recurrent laryngeal nerve	Pancoast syndrome
Brachial plexus	Hemidiaphragmatic paralysis
Pericardium	Effusion
Superior vena cava	Facial swelling
Great vessels	Massive haemoptysis
Oesophagus	Dysphagia

25   GASTRIC CANCER

In which countries is gastric cancer still common?

Far East:

*   Japan
*   China.

Can you describe the epidemiology and pathological features of gastric cancer?

Epidemiology:

*   Second commonest fatal malignancy worldwide
*   UK incidence 3/10,000
*   55–65 years; male:female ratio 2:1
*   Overall 5-year survival rate 10%.

Aetiology/risk factors:

*   Lower social class
*   Associated with nitrate consumption (smoked fish/ spiced foods)
*   Blood group A; pernicious anaemia
*   Atrophic gastritis, benign gastric ulcer.

Location:

*   Pylorus/antrum 50%–60%
*   Cardia 25%
*   Body/fundus 15–25%.

Histology:

*   90% are adenocarcinomas
*   Carcinoid
*   Lymphomas.

What is known about lymphoma of the stomach?

*   Commonest site of gastrointestinal lymphomas
*   Associated with *Helicobacter pylori* infection
*   Gastric mucosal lymphoid tissue resembles MALT (mucosa-associated lymphoid tissue), ie follicles with germinal centres. This tissue forms the basis of B-cell lymphomas.

26   HISTOLOGY AND CYTOLOGY

What is the difference between cytology and histology?

- Both involve the study of cells at the microscopic level.
- **Cytology** studies individual cells and cell morphology.
- **Histology** studies cells within the context of tissues, and provides information about tissue architecture.

Can you give some examples where these techniques are used?

Cytology is usually performed on aspirates of fluids or brushings from epithelial surfaces. Examples include:

- Fine-needle aspiration cytology (thyroid, lymph node, breast disease)
- Bronchial brushings (lung carcinoma)
- Peritoneal aspiration (intra-abdominal malignancy)
- Pleural aspiration (lung and pleural malignancy)
- Urine (bladder malignancy)
- Brushings from endoscopic retrograde cholangiopancreatography (ERCP) (biliary tree and pancreatic malignancy)
- Pap smear (cervical malignancy).

Histology is performed on a tissue specimen, which is obtained by biopsy. Types of biopsy include:

- Endoscopic (cystoscopy in bladder cancer, colonoscopy in colorectal cancer)
- Excisional (breast lumpectomy, colectomy, thyroidectomy, skin lesions)
- Incisional (Trucut biopsy in breast disease, TRUS biopsy in prostate disease)
- Diathermy loop (used in transurethral resection of the prostate (TURP) and transurethral resection of bladder tumour (TURBT); cone biopsy in cervical pathology)
- Punch (skin lesions; epidermis and dermis), intra epithelial neoplasia
- Shave (skin lesions; epidermis only)
- Bone marrow (haematological disorders).

What are the advantages and disadvantages of each technique?

	Cytology	Histology
Procedure	Simple to perform; can be performed by all doctors in both the outpatient and ward settings. Generally minimally invasive	Technically more difficult to perform and may require special conditions, such as an operating theatre and general anaesthetic. Generally invasive
Field	Large, poorly defined field sampled	Small, localised field sampled
Usefulness	Good at diagnosing cancer (but not thyroid follicular cancer)	Good at diagnosing cancer; provides information regarding tissue architecture; provides definitive diagnosis of invasion, so aids in the staging of cancers
Cost	Inexpensive; requires minimal equipment	May be expensive; requires specialised instruments ± operation

27   THROMBOSIS

What is the pathogenesis of postoperative deep vein thrombosis (DVT)?

Virchow's triad:

- Stasis
- Hypercoagulability
- Endothelial damage.

What are the risk factors for postoperative DVT?

- Previous DVT
- Lower limb and hip surgery
- Pelvic surgery
- Pregnancy
- Polycythaemia
- Malignancy
- Oral contraceptive pill (OCP)
- Obesity
- Immobility.

How do you reduce the risk of DVT?

Preoperative measures:

- DVT prophylaxis, eg low molecular weight heparin (LMWH)
- Stopping OCP 1 month prior to surgery.

Intraoperative measures:

- Adequate hydration
- Footpumps (pneumatic calf compression)
- Thromboembolic deterrent (TED) stockings.

Postoperative measures:

- Early mobilisation
- Prophylactic LMWH
- TED stockings.

28   ANEURYSM

What is the definition of an aneurysm?

Definition: An aneurysm (*aneuruno*, Greek, to widen out) is defined as an abnormal dilatation of a vessel by at least 50%.

This is usually determined by comparison with an adjacent normal part of the vessel.

What complications may be associated with abdominal aortic aneurysm surgery?

Immediate complications:

*   Bleeding
*   Distal embolisation
*   Massive blood transfusion complications
*   Hypotension
*   Death.

Early complications:

*   Bleeding
*   Myocardial infarction
*   Cardiac arrhythmias
*   Respiratory failure
*   Renal failure (acute tubular necrosis)
*   Acute limb ischaemia
*   Colonic ischaemia and ileus
*   Impotence
*   Multiple-organ failure
*   Death.

Late complications:

*   Aortoduodenal fistula
*   False aneurysm
*   Graft infection.

Why is it necessary to warn the anaesthetist before removing the clamp at the end of an abdominal aortic aneurysm repair?

'Clamp shock': Reperfusion of the lower limbs on removal of the clamps results in the release of oxygen-free radicals, carbon dioxide and lactate from the ischaemic lower limbs. This causes vasodilatation and a reduction in systemic vascular resistance, resulting in hypotension.

29   METAPLASIA

What is metaplasia and how does it differ from dysplasia?

Metaplasia is a change of one fully differentiated cell type into another fully differentiated type of cell. **Dysplasia** is the degree of failure of maturation of tissue and is associated with a tendency for aneuploidy and pleiomorphism without the capacity for invasive spread.

How may metaplasia be classified?

Epithelial metaplasia:

- Squamous metaplasia – commonest, eg cervix, bronchus
- Columnar-cell metaplasia – stomach, usually associated with *H. pylori*; Barrett's oesophagus lined by metaplastic intestinal or gastric mucosa.

Connective tissue metaplasia:

- Osseous metaplasia – in bladder, scars, bronchi (tracheopathia osteoplastica)
- Myeloid metaplasia (marrow formation) – in liver, spleen, lymph nodes
- Chondroid metaplasia – in scars.

What is the significance of metaplasia?

- May become dysplastic if the causative agent persists
- May be misdiagnosed clinically/histologically as dysplastic epithelium
- May be misdiagnosed as carcinoma (eg intestinal metaplasia of the oesophagus), with treatment consequences.

30   TETANUS

What is the infective organism in tetanus?

Clostridium tetani, a Gram-positive anaerobic 'drum stick' bacteria from soil.

Describe the mechanism by which tetanus causes problems in humans?

- Toxic proteins are absorbed into motor nerve endings and anterior horn cells.
- Tetanospasmin is neurotoxic, reducing neuromuscular inhibition and causing spasm:
  - extensors > flexors
  - opisthotonus (arched back)
  - masseter (lockjaw) muscle
  - facial (risus sardonicus) muscles
  - (apnoea) diaphragm.
- Tetanolysin causes red blood cell haemolysis.

What are the principles of prevention and treatment?

Identification of at-risk patients with open wounds and tetanus prone features:

- >6 hours old
- Non-linear wounds
- >1 cm deep
- Burns, crush or high-energy wounds
- Contaminated or devitalised wounds – wound toilet required with early and thorough debridement and lavage.

Management:

- Prophylaxis or immunisation as required
- Tetanus toxoid for all patients with full immunisation (3 × 0.5 ml intramuscularly)
- Passive immunisation (500 IU immunoglobulin) for all high-risk patients or those without prior immunisation
- In established tetanus infection, antibiotics and supportive treatment, including paralysis and ventilation, are required.

2

PRINCIPLES OF SURGERY

1   DIATHERMY

How does diathermy work?

- Diathermy works on the principle of passage of high-frequency AC current through body tissue. Where the current is locally concentrated, heat is produced, with temperatures of up to 1000 °C.
- Cell water is instantly vaporised, causing tissue disruption with coagulation of blood vessels.

What is the difference between bipolar and monopolar diathermy?

Monopolar diathermy:

- Uses a high-power unit (400 W).
- The current passes from the active electrode (high current density), which is held by the surgeon.
- The current passes through the body via a patient plate electrode (low current density).
- The plate electrode should have a contact area of >70 cm^2, good contact with skin, and should be away from bony prominences.

Bipolar diathermy:

- Uses a lower power unit (50 W).
- The current passes down one limb of the forceps, through the tissue and up the other limb.
- There is no need for a patient plate electrode.
- Inherently safer.
- No cutting or 'buzzing' modes.

What are the dangers of using diathermy in patients with cardiac pacemakers and what can you do to avoid these?

The high-frequency diathermy current may interact with the logic circuits in the pacemaker, which can inhibit the pacemaker itself, increase pacing, or even cause reprogramming.

Diathermy close to the pacemaker box may result in current travelling down the pacing wire, causing a myocardial burn. The resultant effects range from affecting the threshold potential to cardiac arrest.

Safety considerations when using diathermy:

- Contact the cardiologist – the patient may need re-programming of their pacemaker pre- and postoperatively.
- Use bipolar diathermy if possible.
- If monopolar diathermy is needed, use short bursts at the lowest power possible. The patient pad should be placed as far away from the active electrode as possible and in a way that directs current away from the pacemaker.

2 STERILISATION

What is the difference between disinfection and sterilisation?

Disinfection is the reduction in the number of viable micro-organisms. **Sterilisation** is the complete destruction of all viable micro-organisms, including spores, cysts and viruses.

What methods of sterilisation do you know of?

There are physical and chemical methods of sterilisation.

Physical methods:

- **Moist heat** (autoclave) – saturated steam at high pressure, 134 °C at 30 lb/in^2 for 3 minutes (holding time), or 121 °C at 15 lb/in^2 for 15 minutes.
- **Dry heat** – hot-air ovens, for moisture-sensitive equipment, eg non-stainless steel instruments, instruments with fine cutting edges. Effective but inefficient, requiring 160 °C for at least 2 hours.
- **Irradiation** – γ irradiation, used for sterilisation of large batches of equipment on an industrial scale, commonly for single-use items.
- **Filtration** – for heat-labile liquids, dependent on pore size. Used to sterilise drugs for injection.

Chemical methods:

- **Ethylene oxide** – highly penetrative agent, effective at ambient temperatures and pressures. Used for heat-labile articles. Good for electrical equipment, rubber, plastics. It is, however, highly explosive, toxic, irritant and carcinogenic. Mainly used for industrial processes.
- **Formaldehyde** – dry saturated steam in combination with formaldehyde, using low temperatures (73 °C for 2 hours). Good for heat-labile equipment, but not used on items contaminated with body fluids as proteins are fixed and deposited on equipment.

What methods are used to monitor the efficacy of sterilisation?

- **Brownes tubes** – bottles containing indicator solution, placed amongst equipment to be sterilised. It changes colour from red to green after adequate heat sterilisation.
- **Bowie-Dick test** – heat-sensitive ink present on special tape. Stripes on the tape change colour to a darker brown when equipment has been adequately sterilised.

3   DIABETIC SURGICAL PATIENT

How do you classify diabetes mellitus?

Primary: genetic, infective, immunological.
Secondary: pancreatic disease, insulin antagonism (steroids), drugs.

Or:

Type 1 diabetes: insulin-dependent.
Type 2 diabetes: non-insulin-dependent; diet-controlled or requires oral hypoglycaemic drugs.
Diagnosis: random plasma glucose >11 mmol/l or fasting glucose >8 mmol/l.

How do you assess diabetic control and how does diabetes affect the body?

Diabetic control:

- History, eg of hypoglycaemic episodes, fatigue, weight loss, thirst, excessive urination
- Glycosylated haemoglobin (HbA_{1c}) levels (normal levels are 3.8%–6.4%; >9% indicates poor control).

Systems affected by diabetes mellitus:

- Peripheral nervous system – autonomic and peripheral neuropathy, eg hypotension, sexual dysfunction, bladder dysfunction, faecal incontinence, constipation, gastroparesis
- Cardiovascular system – ischaemic heart disease, cerebrovascular disease, cardiomyopathy
- Peripheral vascular system – leg ulceration, claudication
- Renal system – diabetic nephropathy, end-stage renal disease
- Eye disease – retinopathy, cataract, glaucoma.

Why is tight control of glucose so important?

Hyperglycaemia causes:

- Osmotic diuresis
- Dehydration
- Hyperosmolarity
- Hyperviscosity of blood and predisposition to thrombosis
- Cerebral oedema
- Increased risk of wound infection.

All these lead to increased complication rates and prolonged hospital stay.

4   PRINCIPLES OF FRACTURE MANAGEMENT

What is a fracture?
A break in the structural continuity of the cortex of bone, with associated soft-tissue injury.

What are the processes involved in fracture healing?

- **Haematoma formation** – devitalised bone dies back
- **Inflammation and cellular proliferation** – haematoma organises to form granulation tissue
- **Callus formation** – cellular soft callus, derived from periosteal cells, creating woven bone
- **Consolidation** – continued osteoblastic and osteoclastic action, converting woven bone to lamellar bone
- **Remodelling** – callus remodels according to stresses in the bone.

How do you treat fractures?

Principles: reduce and hold the fracture in a satisfactory position until union has occurred, followed by early mobilisation.

Reduction:

- Closed
- Open.

Immobilisation:

- Non-operative:
  - traction: skeletal/skin
  - cast splintage: plaster of Paris, synthetic materials
  - other forms of splintage, eg neighbour strapping, finger splints
- Operative:
  - internal fixation: plates, screws, K-wires, intramedullary nailing
  - external fixation: uniplanar, biplanar, circular (Ilizarov), hybrid.

Early mobilisation:

- Mobilise uninvolved joints in the same limb as soon as possible to prevent stiffness.
- Cast bracing can be used to improve stability of a partially united fracture to help early mobilisation (eg tibial plateau fracture).

5   SUTURES

What types of suture material do you know of?

Non-absorbable:

- Silk
- Nylon, eg Ethilon®, Dermalon®
- Polyester, eg Ticron®
- Polypropylene, eg Surgilene®, Prolene®
- Steel wire
- Polytetrafluoroethylene, eg GoreTex®.

Absorbable:

- Polyglycolic acid, eg Dexon®
- Polyglyconate, eg Maxon®
- Polyglactin 910 (Vicryl®)
- Polydioxanone (PDS)
- Polyglecaprone (Monocryl®).

By what mechanisms are sutures absorbed?

- Proteolytic digestion
- Hydrolysis.

What characteristics would the ideal surgical suture have?

- All-purpose, ie can be used for all types of surgery
- Easy to handle
- No memory
- Minimally reactive with tissue, with no predisposition to bacterial growth
- Capable of holding tissue layers throughout the critical wound healing period
- Holds securely when knotted, without fraying or cutting
- Resistant to shrinking in tissues
- Absorbed completely with minimal tissue reaction after serving its purpose
- Non-carcinogenic
- Cheap.

6   GUNSHOT WOUNDS

How would you classify gunshot wounds?

The injury inflicted by a projectile is dependent mainly on its velocity:

Kinetic energy $= \frac{1}{2}mv^2$

Gunshot wounds can be broadly divided into those caused by **low-velocity** (energy) and **high-velocity** (energy) projectiles. High-velocity projectiles induce temporary cavities, up to 30 times the size of the projectile. This causes extensive tissue damage well away from the track, sucking in debris and bacteria on collapsing.

Some bullets flatten on impact, increasing their cross-sectional area, leading to more rapid deceleration and greater transfer of kinetic energy. Other bullets are designed to fragment on impact, extending the tissue damage.

How can you tell the difference between an entry wound and an exit wound?

Entry wounds usually lie against the underlying tissue due to the direction of the shock wave on impact. The exit wound is not supported by the subcutaneous tissue.

Entry wounds are usually well-defined and round or oval-shaped, with a surrounding 1- to 2-mm blackened area of burn or abrasion at the periphery of the wound.

Exit wounds are usually ragged as result of tissue tearing, having an irregular or 'stellate' appearance.

How would you treat an isolated gunshot wound to the thigh?

- Resuscitate the patient according to ATLS (acute trauma life support) protocols
- Apply direct pressure to any bleeding point
- Crossmatch 4 units of blood
- Administer intravenous antibiotics
- Tetanus prophylaxis
- Analgesia
- Assess neurovascular status of the limb
- Photograph and keep wound covered with dressing soaked in Betadine®.

Further management would involve treatment of the vascular system, bone and soft tissues. This would include:

- Thorough washout, debridement and excision of necrotic tissue
- Delayed closure – may need plastic surgery if a large defect

- May need vascular grafting, nerve grafting
- Stabilisation of fractures.

The 'Mangled Extremity Severity Score' provides a guide to the viability of the limb.

7   THEATRE DESIGN

What is the ideal location for a hospital operating theatre suite?

- Away from the main entrance
- Away from any traffic (ie not on the ground floor)
- Next to the Intensive Therapy Unit (ITU)
- All theatres next to each other (therefore less movement of staff and equipment)
- Close to surgical wards
- Next to Sterile Supply Unit
- Easy route from the Emergency Department for emergency surgery (and also near the Radiology Department).

What are the features of an operating theatre that promote a sterile environment?

- 'Zoning' of the theatre, ie outer zone (offices), restricted-access zone (all staff dressed in "greens", including scrub and anaesthetic rooms), and operating zone (where numbers are kept to an absolute minimum)
- Laminar air flow – air is pumped into theatre through vents in the walls (20–40 air changes per hour)
- Wearing disposable operating garments – bacteria pass more easily through wet, re-usable garments than they do through disposable ones
- Skin preparation using non-spirit-based solutions (eg Betadine®)
- Shaving as close to the time of surgery as possible
- Proper scrubbing technique
- Operating suit.

What are the principles behind an operating tent?

- Particularly relevant for orthopaedic surgery
- High vertical laminar flow in a marked area within the theatre
- Clean air from above the table is pumped out through a funnel shape below the table
- Up to 600 changes of air per hour (normal is 20–40/hour).

8   SURGICAL INFECTION

How do you classify surgical wounds?

- **Clean** – no entry into respiratory, genitourinary or gastrointestinal systems (postoperative infection rate should be <2%)
- **Clean-contaminated** – opposite to the above (5% infection rate)
- **Contaminated** – acute inflammation found at surgery but no pus (20% infection rate)
- **Dirty** – pus found at operation (40% infection rate).

What technical surgical factors increase postoperative infection rates?

- Increased duration of surgery
- Rough or careless handling of tissues
- Ligating large tissue pedicles
- Over-thick ligatures
- Haematoma
- Necrotic or ischaemic tissue
- Insertion of a drain through the wound.

When should prophylactic antibiotics be used?

Prophylactic antibiotics should be used:

- When there is an increased risk of infection
- When a graft or implant is used
- In patients with valvular heart disease (infective endocarditis prophylaxis).

Administer antibiotics at the time of induction of anaesthesia and repeat dose at 4–6 hours if the operation is prolonged.

9 WOUND DEHISCENCE

What may be the result of failure of a wound to heal?

- Superficial wound disruption
- Wound dehiscence
- Incisional hernia.

What are the risk factors for wound dehiscence?

The main risk factor is **technical surgical error**. There are, however, other factors that play a role.

Preoperative factors:

- Respiratory disease
- Smoking
- Jaundice
- Chronic obstructive pulmonary disease
- Protein deficiency
- Steroids
- Malignant disease.

Intraoperative (ie surgical) factors:

- Inadequate evacuation of pus, haematoma, slough and any foreign body
- Tissues sutured under high tension
- Incorrectly placed sutures.

Postoperative factors:

- Infection
- Persistent cough.

How is an abdominal wound dehiscence managed?

- Resuscitation of the patient
- Application of a sterile Betadine® gauze pack over the wound (and bowel if eviscerated)
- Urgent re-exploration of abdomen
- Copious peritoneal lavage
- Resuture of the wound with non-absorbable suture material.

10   CONSENT

What is informed consent?

Making a considered choice about **a treatment or procedure after sufficient appreciation of the pertinent facts** that is in the individual patient's best interests, balancing the views of the doctor with their own opinions, values and beliefs.

The doctor's role is to:

*   Describe the procedure itself, including the prognosis
*   Discuss risks and complications
*   Offer alternatives where available.

Why does one obtain consent from a patient for a general anaesthetic but not for venepuncture?

Implied verbal consent is adequate for simple procedures and for routine physical examination.

Note that a signed consent form does not give legal proof of the patient having consented, but implies that some degree of discussion has taken place.

What is 'Gillick competence'?

This relates to an anomaly in the consenting of children in that they can only agree to treatment after the age of 18 years but can refuse it from the age of 16 years. The Gillick competence is a legal term which means that if the child (under 16 years) can understand the significance of the treatment, they **can** consent to treatment without their parents or legal guardian consenting on their behalf. In practice, it is a situation that should be avoided if at all possible.

11   CHRONIC OBSTRUCTIVE PULMONARY DISEASE

When would you suspect that a patient has chronic obstructive pulmonary disease (COPD)?

If the patient has a cough, producing sputum on most days for 3 months of the year for two consecutive years.

What steps should you take in the preparation of a patient with COPD for theatre?

- Emphasise the importance of stopping smoking.
- Speak to the anaesthetist beforehand and organise a respiratory consultant opinion. Discuss the need for post-op ventilation.
- These patients often need preoperative lung function tests and optimisation of current therapy.
- Book the procedure in the summer months if possible.
- Consent issues – important to mention all pertinent risks.

How is the patient managed postoperatively?

- Multidisciplinary approach (eg anaesthetist, respiratory physician, physiotherapist)
- May require postoperative ventilation in an ITU or High Dependency Unit (HDU)
- Early intensive physiotherapy
- Sitting the patient upright
- Discharge planning as soon as possible to prevent postoperative infections.

12   OUTCOMES OF SURGERY

What do you understand by the term 'outcomes', with respect to surgery?

Defined as the result of clinical intervention and may represent success or failure of a procedure. It can be measured in terms of:

- Surgical mortality
- Complication rates
- Patient satisfaction
- Length of hospital stay
- Quality of life.

How can the benefits of surgical treatment be measured economically?

Economic measurements are quite difficult to make, but cost effectiveness can be assessed in terms of:

- Cost savings or avoidance of unnecessary costs (eg reducing smoking)
- Effective improvement in patient care.

Benefits can therefore be measured by:

- Cure
- Increased life expectancy
- Increased quality of life.

What is a 'quality-adjusted life year' (QALY) and how is it defined?

One QALY is the value of a healthy life measured in years, that is one full-quality year of life is one QALY. Two 6-month periods over 2 years in full health is also defined as one QALY.

13   LOCAL ANAESTHESIA

How do local anaesthetic agents work?

Most local anaesthetic agents are reversible membrane-stabilising drugs, occupying sodium channels in the axon membrane, so preventing the passage of sodium ions and the propagation of action potentials.

What precautions and maximum doses apply to local anaesthetic infiltration?

- Implied or written consent
- Precautionary intravenous access
- Avoidance of intravascular injection
- Availability of resuscitation equipment
- Monitoring of patients for 30 minutes post-infiltration.

Lidocaine maximum dose:

4 mg/kg plain 1% lidocaine, ie 28 ml (280 mg) for a 70-kg patient
7 mg/kg 1% lidocaine with adrenaline, ie 50 ml (500 mg) for a 70-kg patient
(1% lidocaine = 10 mg/ml; low-concentration adrenaline is used – 1:200,000)

Bupivacaine maximum dose:

2.5 mg/kg plain 0.25% bupivacaine, ie 70 ml for a 70-kg patient (or 35 ml of 0.5% bupivacaine)
3.2 mg/kg 0.25% bupivacaine with adrenaline, ie 90 ml for a 70-kg patient (or 45 ml of 0.5% bupivacaine + adrenaline)
(0.25% bupivacaine = 2.5 mg/ml; adrenaline, 1:200,000)

What are the toxic effects of local anaesthetics and how do you manage them?

Local anaesthetic toxicity occurs in two main forms:

1   **Central nervous system toxicity**, classically said to occur in three phases:
    - excitation pase – tinnitus, confusion, circumoral tingling, light-headedness
    - convulsive phase – grand mal seizure
    - central nervous system (CNS) depression – drowsiness, collapse, coma, apnoea.
2   **Cardiovascular system toxicity:**
    - excitation phase – hypertension, tachycardia
    - cardiovascular depresssion – hypotension
    - cardiovascular collapse.

Management of local anaesthetic toxicity:

- Airway support with oxygen administration
- Establish intravenous access
- Anticonvulsant agents (diazepam, thiopentone) and cardiopulmonary resuscitation (adrenaline).

14   NEEDLES

What are the various parts of a needle called?

- Point
- Body
- Swage (attachment to the suture).

What are the important characteristics of suture needles in surgery?

- The type of needle is determined by the procedure, the tissue, access, gauge of the suture and surgeon preference.
- Needles are mostly swaged/eyeless (pre-threaded and less traumatic), except Mayo needles.
- Some needles have a flat, grasping section in the body with ribs to prevent rotation.
- Cutting needles have a sharp triangular cross-section with an apex on the inside for tough tissue (skin).
- The body of the needle can be:
  - straight
  - circular, with variable fractions of circumference, eg $3/8$ circle, $1/2$ circle
  - rounded, to separate tissues and create a watertight suture line (gastrointestinal or cardiac).

What types of specialised needles do you know of?

- Increased circumference – for more restricted areas ($5/8$ circle)
- Reverse cutting – with the sharp edge on the outside of the curvature to protect tissue inside
- Blunt taperpoint – to reduce the risk of needlestick injuries
- Blunt point – for suturing friable vascular tissue (eg liver, spleen, kidney)
- Heavy body – for tough tissue
- J-shaped or compound – for specific uses (laparoscopy wound closure or femoral hernia repair).

15 BURNS

What is a burn and how are burns classified?

Definition: A burn is coagulative damage to the surface layers of the body caused by heat, cold, friction, electrical or chemical insults. Burns are classified according to depth:

- **Superficial**/(first-degree)/erythema – heal from basal cells
- **Dermal**/(second-degree)/partial thickness – red, mottled, with blisters; hypersensitive; healing depends on re-epithelialisation from hair follicles, sweat and sebaceous glands
- **Full thickness**/(third-degree) – dark, leathery, painless and dry.

Can you describe the important principles of burns management?

- ATLS (consider inhalational injury and concomitant trauma).
- Assess the size, depth and location of the burn ('rule of nines' or Lund and Bowder chart).
- Cold water irrigation to control pain and prevent further tissue injury.
- Decide between open- and closed-dressing management.
- Calculate fluid requirements using a fixed protocol, eg Muir and Barclay formula.
- Beware of circumferential burns and circulatory compromise needing escharotomy.
- Note that >10% total surface area burns in children/ elderly and >20% total surface area burns in adults will require patient transfer to a regional burns unit.
- Early nutritional supplementation (enteral > parenteral).

What are the complications of a burn injury?

Immediate complications:
- myonecrosis from deep burns (require debridement)
- renal failure – develops unless high urine output maintained (hypovolaemia, haemoglobinuria, high potassium load)
- hypernatraemia (unreplaced fluid) or hyponatraemia and cerebral oedema (hypotonic resuscitation)
- myocardial depression.

Early complications:
- gastrointestinal ulceration (Curling's ulcers) and catabolic state
- infection (pneumonia, central line infection, toxic shock from *Staphylococcus aureus*)
- disseminated intravascular coagulation (from massive burns).

Late complications:
- burn contractures.

16   DRESSINGS

What is the purpose of a wound dressing?

- To absorb excess moisture
- To control skin temperature
- To prevent bacteria entering a wound.

Can you describe some types of wound dressing and their properties?

Dressings may be permeable or impermeable:

1   **Permeable dressings:**
    - alginates (eg Kaltostat®) – forms a highly absorbent gel coating with moisture
    - foam dressings (Allevyn®) – variable absorbency; good secondary covering
    - hydrogel (eg Intrasite® gel) – hydrates wound; facilitates autolytic debridement (some absorption); requires secondary covering.

2   **Impermeable dressings:**
    - hydrocolloid (eg Granuflex®) – impermeable absorbent layer on vapour-permeable film; facilitates rehydration and autolytic debridement; promotes granulation.

3   **Vapour-permeable films:**
    - allow the passage of oxygen, but not water or bacteria
    - suitable for moderate exudates only (not leg ulcers)
    - good as secondary dressings and to protect frail skin.

4   **Low-adherence dressings:**
    - paraffin gauze (Jelonet®) or silicone (Mepitil®).

5   **Odour absorbent dressings:**
    - activated charcoal (Lyofoam®).

Do living organisms have any role in wound care?

Leeches (*Hirudo medicinalis*):

- Synthesise an anticoagulant, a local vasodilator and local anaesthetic, allowing continued bleeding (normally up to 10 hours after the leech has detached).
- Venous circulation usually re-established after 3–4 days.
- Used in plastic and microvascular surgery for the re-establishment of blood flow to poorly functioning grafts.

Maggots:

- Secrete a proteolytic enzyme which digests slough and necrotic tissue into semi-liquid form that can be ingested along with bacteria.

- Eggs of the greenbottle (*Lucilia sercata*) are collected from pigs' livers and chemically sterilised.
- Bottles of 300 larvae are applied onto wounds such as leg ulcers, pressure sores, diabetic ulcers, burns and necrotising fasciitis wounds.

17 TOURNIQUETS

Under what circumstances would a tourniquet be useful in surgery?

- Tourniquets are useful in extremity surgery, when a bloodless field is required.
- They are used in the tourniquet test for identifying the presence of lower limb venous incompetence.
- They are useful for the control of haemorrhage when local pressure has failed (temporary use only).

What precautions should you take when using a tourniquet?

- Tourniquets should not be used in patients with peripheral vascular disease and should be avoided in patients who have risk factors for thrombosis.
- When applying a tourniquet, a well-covered area of the limb should be chosen (avoid joints).
- The limb should be well padded with wool, and the tourniquet should have a width of at least half the limb circumference.
- The limb should be exsanguinated with an Esmarch bandage or rubber Rhys-Davies exsanguinator.
- Pneumatic pressure should be applied up to twice the systolic blood pressure in the lower limb or up to the systolic pressure plus 80 mmHg in the upper limb.
- The maximum time allowed is 2 hours.

What are the complications of tourniquet use?

Immediate complications:

- deflation, causing a bleeding field
- pain if applied for longer than 5 minutes if awake
- cardiovascular collapse when deflated (volume diversion)
- muscle damage
- arterial damage (rare).

Early complications:

- inadequate pressure leading to venous congestion
- skin blistering (especially if there are ridges in the cuff or the skin)
- nerve damage (due to pressure effect, not ischaemia)
- pulmonary embolism (reported).

Late complications:

- post-tourniquet palsy
- nerve damage (due to pressure effect, not ischaemia).

18   DRAINS

What are the uses of drains in surgical practice?

- Nasogastric tube to drain stomach air and fluid contents (to prevent aspiration)
- Chest drains (with an underwater seal to prevent backflow resulting from negative intrathoracic pressures) – to drain pleural space
- Operative wound drains (anticipated fluid collection in a closed space) – to prevent seroma formation, eg following incisional hernia repair or in the pelvis
- Pericardial drain post-coronary artery bypass surgery
- Infected abscess cavity drain (intra-abdominal).

How does the underwater seal work in chest drains?

The underwater seal drainage system requires an airtight system to maintain a subatmospheric intrapleural pressure in a collection chamber. The tube is submerged 1–2 cm under the water to minimise resistance to drainage of air/fluid. Inspiration causes fluid to be drawn up the tube until the water pressure matches the intrathoracic pressure. The chamber should be 100 cm below the chest as subatmospheric pressures up to −80 cmH$_2$O may be produced during obstructed inspiration.

What complications can occur with drains?

Immediate complications:

- trauma at insertion.

Early complications:

- failure to drain adequately (incorrect placement, too small, blocked lumen)
- disconnection or removal postoperatively.

Late complications:

- introduction of infection
- erosion of adjacent tissues
- retained foreign body during difficult removal.

19   SCREENING PROGRAMMES

Do you know of any screening programmes currently available in the UK?

There are currently two major screening programmes running in the UK:

- Breast cancer
- Cervical cancer.

What factors make a good screening programme?

Based on World Health Organisation (WHO) guidelines (Wilson and Jungner, 1968):

1   The condition is an important health problem
2   The natural history is well understood
3   Detectable at an early stage
4   Treatment at an early stage is more beneficial than treatment at a later stage
5   Suitable test for detecting early disease
6   Test acceptable
7   Intervals for repeating the test should be established
8   Adequate health service provision available for the increased workload resulting from the test
9   Risks less than the benefits
10 Costs of screening balanced against the benefits.

What biases are associated with screening?

- **Selection bias** – health-conscious individuals tend to take part in screening programmes
- **Lead time bias** – tumours are picked up earlier, leading to increased survival figures
- **Length time bias** – increase in survival due to detection of slow-growing tumours with a better prognosis
- **Diagnosis bias** – inclusion of 'cases' with pre-invasive conditions which would not have progressed to invasive disease.

20   EPIDEMIOLOGY OF DISEASE

What is the difference between incidence and prevalence?

Incidence is the number of new cases in a defined time period within a defined population.

Prevalence is the total number of cases within a defined population.

What do you understand about the term 'cancer registries' in the UK?

- Population-based cancer registries try to assemble a complete count of all incident cancers from notifications of cancer diagnoses by doctors and health service providers, although there is no absolute requirement to do so.
- In the UK, the cancer registry is based in Southport and is voluntary.
- The system is cross-checked by the use of death certificates. The Office of Population, Censuses and Surveys publish all resulting data.

What epidemiological factors need to be considered before a relationship between cause and effect can be established?

The Bradford Hill criteria (1965):

1   Temporal sequence
2   Strength of association
3   Consistency of association
4   Biological gradient (dose response)
5   Specificity of association
6   Plausibility of association
7   Coherence of association (does not conflict with current evidence)
8   Reversibility
9   Analogy
10   Predictive performance.

21   STATISTICS

What is a *P* value and why is a value of <0.05 most frequently used?

- The strength of the difference recorded in hypothesis testing is called the *P* value.
- When a value of 0.05 is used, it implies that one is 95% confident (in 19 out of 20 cases) that any observed difference in the results is real.
- A false conclusion may still occur in 1 in 20 cases.
- There is no scientific basis as to why this figure of $P < 0.05$ is used.
- In general, the smaller the *P* value, the greater the statistical significance.
- A *P* value of 0.01 means that one is even more confident that the findings are real; a false conclusion will only occur in 1 in 100 cases (99% confidence).

When is a chi-squared test used?

The chi-squared test is another form of significance testing for categorical data. It is used to test for an association between two variables (contingency table).

What is the null hypothesis?

- When using statistical tests it is usual to have a position of truth which is constantly being refuted.
- The null hypothesis is the position of truth; the null hypothesis states that there is no difference between two results.
- If a statistical test rejects the null hypothesis, on the basis of the *P* value which is generated, we can conclude that there is indeed a difference.

22   PAIN RELIEF

What is the 'pain relief ladder'?

- The pain relief ladder is a stepwise approach to controlling pain (WHO).
- Additional drugs are added until pain is fully controlled.
- The first step of the ladder uses non-opioid drugs, such as paracetamol or non-steroidal anti-inflammatory drugs (NSAIDs).
- If this is insufficient to control the pain, then weak opioid drugs, such as codeine, are added.
- In the final step of the ladder, strong opioid drugs are used, such as morphine.

What other drugs can be used in conjunction with the pain relief ladder?

- Anti-emetics to ease nausea and vomiting, particularly with opioid drugs
- Anxiolytics, such as diazepam
- Neurological pain – use drugs such as carbamazepine, amitriptyline or gabapentin
- Steroids, such as prednisolone or dexamethasone, increase the efficacy of analgesia, especially for the terminally ill patient.

What are the goals of treatment in the terminally ill patient?

The aim of terminal care is to provide appropriate relief and support from physical and psychological discomfort when cure is not possible. The important areas are to:

- Provide the patient with as much control over their symptoms as possible
- Keep the patient comfortable
- Help the patient, their families and carers organise their lives and deal with issues and concerns
- Prepare them for death.

23   CLINICAL AUDIT

Why is clinical audit used in the National Health Service?

- Clinical audit is used to monitor the care received by patients and the use of interventions within the NHS.
- By comparing service provision against either local or nationally agreed guidelines, deviation from 'best practice' can be highlighted and clinical standards maintained and improved.
- This allows for improvements to be made within a system, in a non-threatening or judgemental environment.
- The audit cycle allows for continued assessment of that system, once improvements have been implemented. Healthcare managers can be informed of areas which require organisational change and additional investment.
- Both patients and the general public gain confidence in the service provided, knowing that best practice has been ensured.

What is the 'audit cycle'?

- The audit cycle commences with the selection of a suitable topic appropriate to the experience and time constraints of the lead person conducting the audit.
- Standards to be compared should be agreed and the audit planned.
- The next phase is initial data collection and analysis.
- Areas for change are highlighted, changes implemented, and then data re-collected, so completing the audit cycle.
- This cycle can be repeated continuously, to improve standards of care.
- Repeat data collections can also be made several years later, to confirm that high standards have been maintained.

What do you understand by the term 'randomised clinical trial'?

The randomised clinical trial is the most powerful method for the accurate assessment of and comparison between treatment options. The treatment options will usually include the standard treatment or placebo and the new treatment option. Randomisation ensures that each patient has an equal chance of receiving either arm(s) of treatment.

24   SKIN COVER

What techniques are available for covering skin defects?

The reconstructive ladder:

- Primary closure ± undermining of skin
- Local flap
- Skin graft
- Distant flap (free flap).

What is a skin graft and what different types exist?

A graft is tissue transferred without its blood supply. Skin grafts always contain the epidermis and some dermis.

Classification by thickness:

- Split thickness (donor site heals by re-epithelialisation from hair follicles, sweat and sebaceous glands)
- Full thickness (with closure of the donor site) – takes longer to heal but gives a better result.

Classification by donor type:

- Autograft (same person)
- Allograft (same species)
- Xenograft (between species).

What is a skin flap and what different types exist?

A flap is tissue transferred with its own blood supply (via a vascular pedicle). The source may be 'local' or 'free':

Local:

- Random pattern (advancement or Z-plasty)
- Axial (islanded on a pedicle).

Free:

- May be composite (multiple tissue types: muscle, fascia, fat and skin – myofasciocutaneous)
- May contain innervation to skin ± muscle
- Can be transferred to non-vascular areas
- Donor sites include latissimus dorsi, rectus abdominis.

25   MRSA

What is MRSA?

- Methicillin-resistant *Staphlococcus aureus*
- Around since the 1960s – increased in the 1970s and became epidemic in the 1980s
- 17 epidemic strains
- Type 15 in UK hospitals.

What are the factors involved in a patient acquiring MRSA?

Patient factors:

- Abnormal damaged skin – burns, ITU
- Length of stay in hospital
- Previous antibiotic treatment.

Organism factors:

- Virulence – the degree or ability of a pathogenic organism to cause disease.

Carrier factors:

- Number and frequency of exposure to carriers present in the hospital environment.

How is MRSA treated?

Colonisation:

- Treat with topical mupirocin.

Infection:

- Treat with intravenous vancomycin (or other anti-MRSA antibiotic)
- As per individual hospital protocol – in close liaison with microbiologist.

26   GOUT

What is the differential diagnosis in a 50-year-old gentleman with a painful toe?

- Common disorders – trauma, hallux valgus, osteoarthritis
- Crystal deposition disorders – gout, calcium pyrophosphate
- Rheumatoid arthritis
- Infection – cellulitis, septic arthritis
- Neoplasia (rare).

What features would make you think of gout as a diagnosis?

Acute attack:

- Metatarsophalangeal joints of toe commonly involved (also ankle, finger, olecranon)
- Skin nodules (tophi)
- Hyperuricaemia, negatively birefringent crystals in synovial fluid on polarised light microscopy.

Chronic attack:

- Recurrent attacks merging into polyarthritis
- Ulceration with chalky discharge
- Renal problems (calculi or parenchymal disease).

How is the diagnosis confirmed and what treatment should be commenced?

Investigations:

- Blood tests – including full blood count (FBC), erythrocyte sedimentation rate (ESR), C-reactive protein
- Joint culture and joint aspiration for microscopy, culture and sensitivity, to exclude infection and birefringency under polarised light ± synovial biopsy
- X-ray – periarticular erosions, normal joint space, soft-tissue swelling; chondrocalcinosis in articular cartilage is indicative of chronic calcinosis, seen in pseudogout.

Treatment:

- Rest
- Anti-inflammatory analgesia (eg indometacin)
- Weight loss and alcohol reduction
- Reduce diuretics
- Uricosuric drugs (allopurinol)
- Colchicine.

27   INFLAMMATORY POLYARTHRITIDES

What causes of polyarthritis do you know?

- Rheumatoid arthritis, osteoarthritis
- Spondyloarthritides – psoriatic arthritis, juvenile idiopathic arthritis, systemic lupus erythematosus (SLE), ankylosing spondylitis, Reiter's syndrome (with urethritis and conjunctivitis)
- Crystal deposition disorders – gout, pseudogout
- Other medical causes, eg Henoch-Schönlein purpura
- Viruses – mumps, rubella, Epstein–Barr virus, hepatitis B virus, enteroviruses, human immunodeficiency virus (HIV).

What are the stages seen in rheumatoid arthritis?

- **Synovitis** – swelling, warmth; affects tendon sheaths and synovium
- **Destruction** – reduced range of movements, tendon ruptures, nodules over elbows (pathognomonic of rheumatoid arthritis)
- **Deformity** – ulnar drift, dislocation of metacarpophalangeal (MCP) joints, fixed flexion deformity of the elbow.

Systemic features include vasculitis and peripheral neuropathy.

How do you distinguish rheumatoid arthritis from osteoarthritis?

	Rheumatoid arthritis	Osteoarthritis
Clinical features	Symmetrical polyarthropathy Symmetrical involvement of proximal interphalangeal joints Subarticular nodules	Asymmetrical monoarthropathy Hypertrophic distal interphalangeal joints
Radiological features	Erosive arthritis	Osteophyte formation Periarticular sclerosis

28 RENAL TRAUMA

Following abdominal trauma, what findings would suggest a renal injury?

- Flank bruising
- Macroscopic haematuria
- Microscopic haematuria associated with hypotension.

How are renal injuries treated?

With increasing use of computed tomography (CT), more patients with both blunt and penetrating renal injuries can be managed non-operatively. Stable haematomas and minimal extravasation can be managed non-operatively.

Indications for operative exploration of the retroperitoneum in patients with penetrating trauma:

- Haemodynamically unstable patient owing to major renal injury; may require a nephrectomy
- Expanding haematoma over the lateral retroperitoneal area or a patient who remains hypotensive despite having no other injuries.

Lesser degrees of renal trauma **should be left well alone**.

The indications for operative exploration in patients with blunt trauma are more controversial:

- Large renal lacerations and extravasation
- Renal pedicle injuries.

How may renal trauma be classified?

Grade*	Type of injury	Description of injury
I	Contusion Haematoma	Microscopic or gross haematuria; urological studies normal Subcapsular, non-expanding without parenchymal laceration
II	Haematoma Laceration	Non-expanding perirenal haematoma confined to renal retroperitoneum <1.0 cm parenchymal depth of renal cortex without urinary extravasation
III	Laceration	>1.0 cm parenchymal depth of renal cortex without collecting system rupture or urinary extravasation
IV	Laceration Vascular	Parenchymal laceration extending through renal cortex, medulla and collecting system Main renal artery or vein injury with contained haemorrhage
V	Laceration Vascular	Completely shattered kidney Avulsion of renal hilum which devascularises kidney

* Advance one grade for bilateral injuries up to grade III.

29   RIB FRACTURES AND PAIN CONTROL

How would you manage an uncomplicated rib fracture?

History:

- Asking about the events that caused the rib fracture can give an idea of the severity of the injury.
- Ask about shortness of breath and haemoptysis.
- Obtain any history of chronic pulmonary problems or heavy smoking.

Examination:

- Palpate for point tenderness and crepitus.
- Examine the patient for possible associated injuries, eg the abdomen for any signs of splenic or hepatic injury.

Investigations: Send the patient for postero-anterior and lateral chest X-rays to exclude pneumothorax, haemothorax or pulmonary contusion.

Management (in the absence of any underlying injury but in the presence of a rib fracture):

- Regular analgesia
- Instruct the patient on the importance of deep breathing and coughing to help prevent pneumonia.
- Inform the patient to expect gradually decreasing discomfort for about 2 weeks, and advise them to avoid strenuous activity for approximately 8 weeks
- Advise the patient to return if there is severe worsening of chest pain, shortness of breath, fever or purulent sputum.

Consider hospitalisation if:

- The patient is elderly
- There is evidence of pulmonary or cardiac compromise
- There are multiple fractures or other injuries.

What are the options for pain control?

These are based on the WHO three-step pain ladder:

Step 1: non-opioids (paracetamol, NSAIDs such as diclofenac)
Step 2: mild opioids (codeine) ± non-opioids
Step 3: strong opioids (morphine; can be given orally, via injection every 3–6 hours or as patient-controlled analgesia) ± non-opioids.

What complications may be encountered with rib fractures?

These depend on the level of the rib fractured.

First rib fracture – usually a sign of major trauma:

- Brachial plexus injury
- Horner's syndrome
- Subclavian artery injury
- Late-developing post-traumatic thoracic outlet syndrome.

Second rib to eighth rib fractures:

- Pneumothorax
- Pleural effusion
- Haemothorax
- Pulmonary contusion
- Pneumonia
- Pulmonary embolus.

Ninth rib to twelfth rib fractures:

- Liver lacerations
- Splenic injury.

30   PROSTATE-SPECIFIC ANTIGEN

What is prostate-specific antigen (PSA), and how is it used clinically?

- Produced by normal and malignant prostate epithelial cells
- Serine protease associated with semen
- PSA is elevated in most patients with:
  - prostatic carcinoma
  - benign prostatic hyperplasia
  - prostatitis
  - post-urinary retention.

PSA is used in combination with digital rectal examination in the management of prostatic carcinoma for:

- Diagnosis
- Follow-up
- Assessment of response to treatment (4 ng/ml is the 'magic' number).

PSA velocity – >0.75 ng/ml/year is associated with prostatic carcinoma.

Prostatic carcinoma is associated with a lower free to total PSA ratio.

Would PSA be a good screening test for prostate cancer?

Yes:

- Common disease
- Major health problem
- Sensitive
- Potential for cure if disease picked up early.

No:

- Not specific
- High number of transrectal ultrasound biopsies
- Poorly defined clinical outcome
- Best treatment for early disease unknown, although there is potential for cure.

What are the different zones of the prostate gland, and what is the pathological significance of these?

Peripheral zone ('left and right lobes'):

- Accounts for 70% of volume in the young prostate
- Most prostatic carcinoma occurs here.

Central zone:

- Accounts for 25% volume.

Transition zone ('middle lobe'):

- Accounts for 5% of volume
- Most benign prostatic hyperplasia occurs here.

3

APPLIED
ANATOMY

1   BREAST

What is the blood supply to the breast?

- Branches of the lateral thoracic artery around and through pectoralis major
- Intercostal perforating branches (especially second and third) from the internal thoracic artery
- Small perforating branches from the posterior intercostal arteries
- Pectoral branches of the thoracoacromial artery (upper breast).

Can you describe the lymphatic drainage of the breast?

- Axillary lymph nodes (75% of lymphatic drainage) – mostly anterior but some direct to central or apical
- Parasternal nodes – along internal thoracic artery
- Posterior intercostal nodes
- Minor pathways (important in malignancy):
  - superficial to opposite breast and anterior abdominal wall
  - supraclavicular and posterior mediastinal.

What nerves are at risk when performing an axillary clearance?

- Thoracodorsal nerve to latissimus dorsi (C6, C7, C8) on posterior axillary wall
- Long thoracic nerve (to serratus anterior), just behind mid-axillary line on medial wall
- Lateral branch of the second intercostal nerve (intercostobrachial nerve) – sensation to medial arm
- Medial and lateral pectoral nerves to pectoralis major and minor (especially in a level 3 clearance).

2   MALE URETHRA

What are the indications for male urethral catheterisation?

- Infravesical obstruction (benign prostatic hyperplasia, haematuria, stricture, inflammation)
- Monitoring of urine output
- Following lower urinary tract surgery
- Neuropathic bladder drainage
- Investigations (urodynamics, cystogram)
- Urine collection.

How is male urethral catheterisation performed?

- Confirm indication via history and examination.
- Explain the procedure to the patient.
- Administer antibiotic prophylaxis.
- Equipment needed:
  - sterile pack
  - catheter
  - antiseptic
  - swabs
  - lidocaine gel
  - urine bag
  - syringe and saline.
- Retract foreskin and prepare site; inject gel; use 'clean' hand to insert catheter; inflate after urine drains.
- Replace foreskin (to prevent paraphimosis).
- Send urine for microscopy, culture and sensitivity.

Describe the anatomy of the male urethra, including potential sites of obstruction.

From distal to proximal:

- Urethral meatus
- Fossa navicularis
- Penile, spongy, membranous and prostatic urethra
- Bladder neck.

Site of obstruction varies according to age:

- In the young, the urethra obstructs at the external sphincter.
- In older men, the urethra obstructs at prostate/bladder neck.

3   SCALP

Can you name the layers of the scalp?

From superficial to deep, using the mnemonic SCALP:

- **S**kin
- Dense **C**onnective tissue
- Galea **A**poneurosis
- **L**oose areolar tissue
- **P**ericranium (periosteum of the skull).

What is the depth of injury seen in a gaping scalp laceration? What are the resultant risks?

Deep injuries:

- In a gaping scalp wound, the galea aponeurosis has been breached.
- The galea and pericranium slide over one another easily through the loose areolar tissue.

Superficial injuries:

- The outer three layers are firmly bound to each other, so superficial lacerations do not gape.

There is an increased **risk of infection** if the potential space between the galea and pericranium is exposed, with possible intracranial sepsis ensuing.

Why does the scalp bleed so profusely when injured?

The scalp is highly vascularised and has a rich anastomotic network. The blood supply includes:

- **External carotid artery:**
  - superficial temporal artery
  - posterior auricular artery
  - occipital artery

- **Internal carotid artery:**
  - ophthalmic artery via the supraorbital artery.

4   HIP JOINT

What type of joint is the hip joint?

- The hip joint is a synovial ball and socket joint lined by hyaline articular cartilage.
- The acetabulum is deepened by the labrum (triangular in section). "
- The acetabulum is horseshoe-shaped, with a central pad of fat (Haversian pad), with an inferior margin marked by the transverse acetabular ligament.
- The femoral head is two-thirds of a sphere; the ligamentum teres attaches at the fovea capitis.

What is the blood supply to the hip joint?

The **trochanteric anastomosis (extracapsular arterial ring)** is the main source of blood supply to the femoral head and intracapsular neck. Branches run along the femoral neck as ascending cervical branches with the retinacular fibres of the capsule. Formed by anastomosis of descending branch of the superior gluteal artery with ascending branches of lateral and medial circumflex arteries (LFCA and MFCA); the inferior gluteal artery usually joins the anastomosis.

Note that there is also a **cruciate anastomosis** at the level of the lesser trochanter formed by MFCA, LFCA, an ascending branch of the first perforator artery and descending branch of the inferior gluteal artery.

The **artery of ligamentum teres** is derived from the obturator artery or MFCA. It is usually atrophied by the age of 7 years, but can bleed during surgery in the adult.

Epiphyseal blood supply – arises from lateral epiphyseal vessels of the subsynovial arterial ring (found at the articular cartilage-neck junction) and enters the head posterosuperiorly.

Metaphyseal blood supply – arises from the extracapsular arterial ring.

What conditions can compromise the blood supply to the femoral head?

- Fractures – especially intracapsular fractures of the femoral neck
- Dislocations – most commonly posterior, from dashboard injury following road traffic accidents (RTA)
- Drugs, eg steroids, alcohol
- Metabolic, eg gout, diabetes
- Hereditary, eg sickle cell anaemia, Gaucher's disease
- Developmental, eg Perthes, slipped upper femoral epiphysis (SUFE)
- Miscellaneous, eg Caisson disease, pregnancy, renal transplant.

5   SCIATIC NERVE

**What is the course of the
sciatic nerve?**

- Roots L4, L5, S1, S2, S3
- Largest branch of the sacral plexus (which lies on the
  fromt of piriformis), formed at the lower margin of
  piriformis by the union of tibial and common peroneal
  parts
- Lies on ischium, over posterior part of acetabulum
  at a point a third of the way up from from the ischial
  tuberosity to the posterior superior iliac spine (PSIS; the
  surface marking for entry into gluteal region)
- Lies under cover of gluteus maximus in the buttock,
  midway between the greater trochanter and the ischial
  tuberosity
- Passes vertically down over the posterior surface
  of obturator internus and quadratus femoris to the
  hamstring compartment of the thigh, lying on adductor
  magnus where it is crossed posteriorly by long head of
  biceps femoris
- Divides into the common peroneal nerve (L4, L5, S1,
  S2) and the tibial nerve (L4, L5, S1, S2, S3) in the upper
  part of politeal fossa. (There may be a high division
  where the two parts leave separately from pelvis, with
  the common peroneal nerve piercing piriformis and the
  tibial nerve emerging beneath it)
- All muscle branches come from the medial side of the
  sciatic nerve except for the short head of biceps – so
  lateral side is the side of relative safety for exposure.

**What is the clinical
manifestation of damage to
the sciatic nerve?**

Motor:

- Above knee – paralysis of hamstrings
- Below knee – paralysis of all muscles of the leg and
  foot, with foot drop deformity.

Sensory:

- Below knee – complete loss of sensation, except for
  area supplied by the saphenous branch of the femoral
  nerve (medial side of leg, medial malleolus and medial
  aspect of foot down to the midfoot).

**Where is the safe zone for
giving an intramuscular
injection in the buttock?**

The safe zone where a needle can enter gluteus minimus
or maximus is the area covering an outstretched hand on
the buttock, with the tip of the thumb and thenar eminence
touching the anterior superior iliac spine.

6   POPLITEAL FOSSA

What are the boundaries of the popliteal fossa?

The popliteal fossa is a rhomboid-shaped space behind the knee. The boundaries are summarised below:

Superolateral	Biceps femoris
Superomedial	Semitendinosus and semimembranosus
Inferolateral	Lateral head of gastrocnemius
Inferomedial	Medial head of gastrocnemius
Roof	Fascia lata (pierced by short saphenous vein and posterior femoral cutaneous nerve)
Floor	From above down: • Popliteal surface of femur • Posterior aspect of knee joint capsule reinforced by oblique popliteal ligament • Popliteus muscle (popliteus is intracapsular from triangular area on posterior surface of tibia above the soleal line; it runs superolaterally to attach to the lateral surface of the lateral condyle of the femur, lateral meniscus and capsule – supplied by the tibial nerve and acts to unlock the knee at the start of flexion)

What are the contents of the popliteal fossa?

- From superficial to deep: nerves, vein, then artery.
- The common peroneal nerve leaves the fossa along the medial border of the biceps tendon and disappears into the substance of peroneus longus (branches in fossa are sural communicating nerve, lateral cutaneous nerve of calf, and superior, inferior and recurrent genicular nerves).
- The tibial nerve lies at first lateral to the popliteal vessels, and then crosses superficially to these vessels to lie on their medial side (motor branches to all muscles in the popliteal fossa – plantaris, both heads of gastrocnemius, soleus and popliteus; sensory – sural).
- The popliteal vein lies superficial to the popliteal artery.
- The fossa also contains fat and popliteal lymph nodes.

What is the differential diagnosis of a swelling in the popliteal fossa?

Skin and soft tissues – lipoma, sebaceous cyst, sarcoma.
Vein – saphena varix of short saphenous vein junction.
Artery – popliteal artery aneursym.

Lymph nodes.
Bursae – Baker's cyst, semimembranosus bursa, gastrocnemius bursa.
Bones – tumour of distal femur or proximal tibia.

7   EPISTAXIS

What are the common sites of epistaxis?

Trivial bleeds tend to be anterior, from the nasal septum (Little's area).

More severe bleeds are often posterior, arterial, and may present with bleeding from both sides of the nose.

How is a minor epistaxis managed?

Management is along the lines of any haemorrhage situation. Anterior epistaxes may be managed by:

- Direct pressure
- Cautery to bleeding point.

How are more severe epistaxes managed?

- Resuscitation (ABC)
- Correction of blood loss, initially with fluid replacement, then blood products (as required)
- Insertion of a nasal pack
- Examination of the nose under anaesthetic
- Cautery of bleeding point
- Arterial ligation:
  - sphenopalatine artery
  - maxillary artery
  - external carotid artery.

8   VARICOSE VEINS

What is the surface marking of the sapheno-femoral junction and can you name the tributaries of the long saphenous vein at this level?

Surface markings:

- 2–3 cm below and lateral to the pubic tubercle.

Tributaries:

- Superficial inferior epigastric vein
- Deep external pudendal vein
- Superficial external pudendal vein
- Superficial circumflex iliac vein
- Antero-postero-medial thigh veins

What complications should be covered during consent of a patient for high saphenous vein ligation, strip and multiple avulsions?

Immediate complications:

- Bleeding
- Femoral vein injury
- Superficial femoral artery injury
- Nerve injury (common peroneal, sural and saphenous nerves).

Early complications:

- Bleeding
- Bruising
- Wound haematoma
- Wound infection
- Seroma
- Lymph leak
- Deep vein thrombosis (DVT).

Late complications:

- Recurrence.

What are the indications for a preoperative duplex scan in patients undergoing varicose vein surgery and what specific questions should be included on the request form?

Indications:

- Recurrent varicose veins
- Sapheno-popliteal incompetence
- Previous or suspicious of DVT.

Questions on the form:

- Are the deep veins patent?
- Are the deep veins incompetent?
- Sites of superficial venous reflux?
- Anatomical landmark for sapheno-popliteal junction in patients with short saphenous incompetence?

9 LOWER LIMB ARTERIAL TREE

What is the surface marking of the common femoral artery?

Mid-inguinal point (midway between the pubic symphysis and the anterior superior iliac spine).

Describe the arterial blood supply of the lower limb.

Common iliac artery – divides into the external and internal iliac arteries in the pelvis.

External iliac artery – passes under the inguinal ligament and becomes the common femoral artery.

Common femoral artery – divides into the profunda femoris (which supplies the thigh) and the superficial femoral artery.

Superficial femoral artery – has no branches in the thigh; passes through the adductor hiatus to become the popliteal artery.

Popliteal artery – divides into the anterior tibial artery and the tibioperoneal trunk.

Tibioperoneal trunk – divides into the posterior tibial and the peroneal arteries.

Posterior tibial artery – runs behind the medial malleolus.

Anterior tibial artery (which becomes the dorsalis pedis artery beyond the line between the malleoli) – passes onto the dorsum of the foot medial to extensor hallucis longus.

Can you describe what structures you encounter when performing a femoral embolectomy?

- Skin
- Fat
- Scarpa's fascia
- Femoral sheath
- The common femoral artery.

The common femoral artery is dissected from the inguinal ligament to beyond the bifurcation of the common femoral artery. The common femoral, profunda femoris and superficial femoral arteries are then exposed.

10   BLADDER

What is the function of the urinary bladder?

Low-pressure storage and emptying system for urine.

Can you describe the structure and relations of the urinary bladder?

Structure:

- Inverted pyramid
- Posterior = **base**
- Superior = **dome**
- Right and left inferolateral surfaces
- Lowest part = **neck**
- Anterior-superior extremity = **apex**.

Relations:

- Superior = peritoneum
- Posterior = rectovesical pouch (males), vesico-uterine pouch (females)
- Base = ductus deferens (cross to medial side of ureter)
- Bladder neck rests on the upper surface of the prostate
- Posteriorly = seminal vesicles
- In the female, the vagina and cervix are bound to the base of the bladder.

How may the bladder be injured?

Bladder injuries have high association with other abdominal pathology; usually well protected by the bony pelvis.

Blunt injury:

- 90% are associated with pelvic fractures
- Occurs in approximately 10% of pelvic fractures
- May be associated with urethral injury, intra-abdominal and renal injury.

Penetrating injury:

- Usually associated with major abdominal injuries.

Iatrogenic injury:

- Laparoscopy
- During transurethral resection of bladder tumours.

11   CHEST WALL

What structures form the thoracic wall?

Anterior – sternum and costal cartilages
Posterior – thoracic part of the vertebral column
Lateral – ribs and intercostal spaces
Superior – suprapleural membrane
Inferior – diaphragm.

Can you name the structures that lie within a typical intercostal space?

Each space contains three muscle layers and an associated neurovascular bundle:

- **External intercostal muscle:** fibres pass downwards and forwards from the rib above to the rib below. They extend from the vertebrae behind to the costochondral junction in front, where the anterior intercostal membrane replaces muscle.
- **Internal intercostal muscle:** fibres pass downwards and backwards from the sternum to the angles of the ribs where it becomes the posterior intercostal membrane.
- **Innermost intercostal muscle:** incompletely separated from the internal intercostal muscle by the neurovascular bundle. The fibres cross more than one intercostal space and may be incomplete. Anteriorly it has a more distinct fan-shaped portion called **transversus thoracis**.

The nerves and vessels of the thoracic wall lie between the internal and innermost intercostal muscle layers. The neurovascular bundle consists, from above downwards, of vein, artery and nerve.

What are the anatomical features of a typical rib?

Each typical rib has a:

- **Head** – has two facets for articulation with the numerically corresponding vertebral body and that of the vertebra immediately above.
- **Neck** – constricted portion between the head and tubercle.
- **Tubercle** – a prominence on the outer surface of the rib at the junction of the neck and the shaft. It has a smooth facet for articulation with the transverse process of the corresponding vertebra.
- **Shaft/body** – thin, flattened and twisted on its long axis. It has a rounded, smooth superior border and a sharp, thin inferior border that has a 'costal groove' (where the intercostal vessels and nerve lie).
- **Angle** – where the shaft of the rib bends sharply forwards.

12   CORONARY VESSELS

Can you describe the arterial circulation to the heart?

The arterial supply of the heart is provided by the right and left coronary arteries, which arise from the aorta immediately above the aortic valve. They lie in the interventricular and atrioventricular grooves over the surface of the heart, lying within the subepicardial connective tissue.

Describe the origins, courses and major branches of the coronary arteries.

Right coronary artery: arises from the anterior aortic sinus of the ascending aorta. It passes forwards between the pulmonary trunk and right auricle. It descends almost vertically in the right atrioventricular groove. At the inferior border of the heart it continues posteriorly along the atrioventricular groove to anastomose with the left coronary artery. The branches of the right coronary artery:

- Marginal branch, to supply the right ventricle
- Posterior interventricular branch, to supply both ventricles, and anastomoses with the anterior interventricular branch of the left coronary artery in the posterior interventricular groove.

Left coronary artery: usually larger than the right coronary artery and arises from the left posterior aortic sinus of the ascending aorta. The left coronary artery passes forwards between the pulmonary trunk and the left auricle. It then enters the atrioventricular groove and divides into:

- Anterior interventricular branch (left anterior descending branch), which runs downwards to the apex of the heart in the anterior interventricular groove and anastomoses with the posterior interventricular branch of the right coronary artery. This branch of the left coronary artery supplies the right and left ventricles and ventricular septum.
- Circumflex branch, which follows the atrioventricular groove, winds around the left margin of the heart and ends by anastomosing with the right coronary artery. It supplies the left atrium and the left ventricle.

What is the venous drainage of the heart?

The main venous drainage of the heart is via veins which accompany the coronary arteries, which open into the right atrium via the coronary sinus. The coronary sinus lies in the posterior atrioventricular groove and is a continuation of the great cardiac vein, opening into the right atrium to the left of the mouth of the inferior vena cava. The small cardiac vein, middle cardiac vein and oblique vein are tributaries of the coronary sinus.

The rest of the venous return enters the right atrium via the anterior cardiac veins (up to three or four in number) and by small veins that open directly into the heart chambers (venae cordis minimae).

13 DIAPHRAGM

What components make up the diaphragm?

Peripheral muscular part:

- Arises from the margins of the thoracic outlet.
- Muscular fibres are arranged in three parts:
  - vertebral part – from the crura and from the arcuate ligaments
  - costal part – attached to the inner aspect of the lower six ribs and costal cartilages
  - sternal portion – consists of two small slips from the deep surface of the xiphisternum.

Central tendinous part:

- Trefoil in shape and partially fused with the undersurface of the fibrous pericardium.

What openings are found in the diaphragm?

The three main openings are:

1. The **aortic opening** (T12 level): lies between the crura and transmits the abdominal aorta, the thoracic duct and often the azygos vein.
2. The **oesophageal opening** (T10 level): lies between the muscular fibres of the right crus of the diaphragm. It transmits the oesophagus, right and left vagus nerves, oesophageal branches of the left gastric vessels and lymphatics from the lower third of the oesophagus.
3. The **caval opening** (T8 level): lies in the central tendon and transmits the inferior vena cava and terminal branches of the right phrenic nerve.

Other openings:

- The greater, lesser and least splanchnic nerves pierce the crura.
- Sympathetic trunks pass posterior to the medial arcuate ligaments on each side.
- Superior epigastric vessels pass between the sternal and costal origins of the diaphragm on each side.
- Left phrenic nerve pierces the left dome to supply the peritoneum on its underside.
- Neurovascular bundles of the seventh to eleventh intercostal spaces pass into the anterior abdominal wall between muscular slips of the costal origin of the diaphragm.

Can you describe the embryological development of the diaphragm?

The diaphragm is formed by the fusion in the embryo of:

- Septum transversum (forming central tendon).
- Dorsal oesophageal mesentery
- A peripheral rim derived from the body wall
- The pleuroperitoneal membranes, which closes the primitive communication between the pleural and peritoneal cavities.

14   HEART

Which structures form the right, left and inferior borders of the heart?

Right border – formed entirely by the right atrium.

Left border – formed mainly by the left ventricle and partly by the auricular appendage of the left atrium.

Inferior border – formed predominantly by the right ventricle but also by the lower part of the right atrium and the apex of the left ventricle.

Describe the conducting system of the heart and the anatomical locations of its components.

- Cardiac beats are initiated in the sinoatrial (SA) node which is situated in the upper part of the crista terminalis, just to the right of the opening of the superior vena cava into the right atrium.
- Impulses then spread through atrial musculature to reach the atrioventricular (AV) node, which lies in the atrial septum above the opening of the coronary sinus.
- Impulses are then conducted to the ventricles via the atrioventricular bundle (of His). This bundle divides at the junction of the membranous and muscular parts of the interventricular septum into its right and left branches and runs immediately beneath the endocardium.

How does the atrial septum form?

- A partition called the **septum primum** grows downwards from the posterior and superior walls of the primitive common atrium to fuse with the endocardial cushions.
- Before this fusion is complete a hole appears in the upper part of the septum called the **foramen secundum** in the septum primum.
- A second membrane, the **septum secundum**, then develops on the right side of the septum primum but it has a free lower edge which extends low enough to overlap the foramen secundum in the septum primum and hence to close it.
- The two overlapping defects in the septa form the valve-like **foramen ovale** which shunts blood from the right to the left heart in the fetus.

15   LUNGS

Can you describe the lobar arrangement of the right and left lung?

The **right lung** is divided into upper, middle and lower lobes by the oblique and horizontal fissures.

The **left lung** is divided into upper and lower lobes by the oblique fissure. The lingular segment of the upper lobe is equivalent to the right middle lobe.

What is a bronchopulmonary segment and what is its surgical significance?

A bronchopulmonary segment is a subdivision of a lung lobe; each lung comprises ten segments. Each segment is supplied by:

- Segmental bronchus
- Segmental artery
- Segmental vein.

The segments are wedge-shaped, with their apices at the hilum and bases at the lung surface. Each segment is surrounded by connective tissue.

Surgical significance:

- Because it is a structural unit, a diseased segment can be removed with little bleeding or alveolar air leakage if it is excised accurately along its boundaries.
- Intersegmental veins within connective tissue mark these boundaries.

What structure lies most superiorly in the lung root and which structures make impressions over the medial aspect of the left lung?

Superior: The pulmonary artery enters the lung root superior to the main bronchus (which in turn is superior to the pulmonary veins).

Medial: The heart, aortic arch and descending aorta make impressions on the medial aspect of the left lung.

16   MEDIASTINUM

How would you anatomically divide the mediastinum?

- Superior mediastinum
- Inferior mediastinum:
  - anterior mediastinum
  - middle mediastinum
  - posterior mediastinum.

What are the boundaries of the superior mediastinum?

Anterior – manubrium sterni.
Posterior – first four thoracic vertebrae.
Superior – root of the neck.
Inferior – an imaginary line drawn from the angle of Louis to the lower border of the T4 vertebra.

What structures are found within the posterior mediastinum?

- Descending thoracic aorta
- Oesophagus
- Vagus and splanchnic nerves
- Azygos and hemiazygos veins
- Thoracic duct
- Posterior mediastinal lymph nodes.

17   LUMBAR VERTEBRAE

What are the characteristic features of a lumbar vertebra?

- There are no foramina in the transverse processes (compared with cervical vertebrae).
- There are no facets on the sides of the body (compared with thoracic vertebrae).
- The body is large, wider in the lateral plane than in the anteroposterior plane.
- The pedicles are very strong, directed backwards from the upper part of the body.
- The laminae are broad, short, and strong.
- The vertebral foramen is triangular, larger than in the thoracic region, but smaller than in the cervical region.
- The spinous processes are thick, broad, and somewhat quadrilateral.
- The superior and inferior articular processes are well defined, projecting respectively upwards and downwards from the junctions of the pedicles and laminae.
- Transverse processes are long, slender, and horizontal in the upper three lumbar vertebrae and they incline upwards in the lower two; they are situated in front of the articular processes instead of behind them as in the thoracic vertebrae.

What are intervertebral discs and in which direction do they usually prolapse?

They are secondary cartilaginous joints, comprising a central **nucleus pulposus** and a peripheral **annulus fibrosus**. They separate the individual vertebrae, and act as shock absorbers for the axial skeleton during motion.

The most common prolapse is a **posterolateral prolapse**:

- Due to strong posterior longitudinal ligament directly posteriorly.
- Can cause nerve root compression.

Less commonly, there may be a **direct posterior prolapse**:

- Can cause spinal cord or cauda equina compression.

What symptoms and signs would someone with an L5–S1 disc prolapse have?

L5–S1 disc prolapse can cause bilateral L5 or S1 radiculopathy.

L5 radiculopathy:

- May present with pain, and paraesthesia/numbness along the posterolateral aspect of the leg, down to the great toe.
- May have weakness of extensor hallucis longus and of dorsiflexion.

S1 radiculopathy:

- May present with pain, and paraesthesia/numbness along the posterior aspect of the leg, down to the lateral aspect of the heel and foot.
- May have weakness of ankle plantar flexion.
- The ankle jerk may be absent.

18   ADDUCTOR CANAL

What are the boundaries of the adductor canal?

Posterior:

- Adductor longus proximally
- Adductor magnus distally.

Anterolateral:

- Vastus medialis.

Anteromedial:

- Fibrous membrane overlapped by sartorius.

What are the contents of the adductor canal?

1. **Femoral artery:** Enters the adductor canal from the femoral triangle and leaves the canal by entering the popliteal fossa via the adductor hiatus in adductor magnus to become the popliteal artery.

2. **Femoral vein:** Lies posterior to the artery.

3. **Saphenous nerve:**

   - Crosses the femoral artery anteriorly from the lateral to the medial side.
   - Leaves the canal by piercing the fibrous roof.

4. **Nerve to vastus medialis**.

5. **Two divisions of the obturator nerve:**

   - Anterior division gives off branches to subsartorial plexus and femoral artery.
   - Posterior division supplies the knee joint.

What is the clinical significance of the adductor canal?

- It is used to expose and ligate the femoral artery, for example during surgery for popliteal artery aneurysms.
- It also represents the most common site for atherosclerotic changes in the lower limb (at the adductor hiatus).

19 PERITONEAL CAVITY

What is the epiploic foramen and what are its boundaries?

The epiploic foramen, also known as the 'foramen of Winslow', is a vertical opening through which the lesser sac communicates with the greater sac.

Boundaries:

- **Anterior** – right free edge of the lesser omentum, containing portal vein, hepatic artery and bile duct
- **Posterior** – inferior vena cava
- **Superior** – caudate process of the liver
- **Inferior** – first part of duodenum.

What are the clinically important subphrenic spaces?

Right subphrenic space:

- Lies between the right lobe of the liver and the diaphragm
- Collections may occur here from infections of the gallbladder and appendix.

Left subphrenic space:

- Lies between the left lobe of the liver and the diaphragm
- Pus may collect after operations on structures such as the stomach and the spleen.

Right subhepatic space:

- Also known as 'Morrison's pouch'
- Most dependent part in the supine position
- Collections may occur here from infections of the gallbladder and appendix.

Left subhepatic space:

- This is the lesser sac.

Right extraperitoneal space:

- Overlies the bare area of the liver
- Infection may spread here from the liver.

What are the common sites of internal herniation within the peritoneal cavity?

- Lesser sac via the foramen of Winslow
- Paraduodenal fossa
- Retrocaecal fossa
- Intersigmoid fossa.

20   THYROID GLAND

Can you describe the thyroid gland and its fuction?

The thyroid is an endocrine gland located in the neck, enclosed within the pretracheal fascia and covered by the strap muscles. It is made up of:

- Two lateral lobes either side of the thyroid cartilage down to the sixth tracheal ring
- An isthmus that connects the two glands and lies over the trachea at the second ring
- Occasionally also a pyramidal lobe projecting cranially from the isthmus.

The function of the thyroid is the secretion of thyroxine (T4) and triiodothyronine (T3), which are important both in development and in maintenance of the basal metabolic rate. Calcitonin is also secreted by the thyroid (involved in calcium homeostasis).

What is its blood and nerve supply and its lymphatic drainage?

The **arterial supply** to the thyroid gland is via:

- Superior thyroid artery from the external carotid artery
- Inferior thyroid artery from the subclavian artery, via the thyrocervical trunk
- A midline thyroid ima artery from the aortic arch in approximately 10% of people.

The **nerve supply** is sympathetic from the superior, middle and inferior cervical sympathetic ganglia, which reach the gland running on the arteries listed above, and are vasomotor. It also receives a vagal supply via cardiac and laryngeal branches.

The **venous drainage** is via three paired veins:

- Superior thyroid vein – facial or internal jugular vein drainage
- Middle thyroid vein – internal jugular vein drainage
- Inferior thyroid vein – brachiocephalic drainage.

The **lymphatics** run via the pretracheal, paratracheal and prelaryngeal regions to the deep cervical nodes and also to the brachiocephalic nodes.

What nerves are in danger during a thyroidectomy?

The **recurrent laryngeal nerve** is intimately related to the inferior thyroid artery and may be posterior or anterior to it.

The **external branch of the superior laryngeal nerve** is related to the superior thyroid artery and is also at risk during this operation.

21   THE MIDDLE EAR

What are the boundaries of the middle ear?

The middle ear is an air-filled cavity in the petrous temporal bone that has the following boundaries:

- **Lateral** – separating the region from the external auditory meatus is the tympanic membrane and, above it, the squamous temporal bone forms the epitympanic attic.
- **Medial** – separating the region from the inner ear is the round window occluded by the secondary tympanic membrane, the oval window filled by the base of the stapes. This wall exhibits two mounds, the promontory of the first turn of the cochlea and the prominence of the facial nerve running past this wall.
- **Superior** – separating the region from the middle cranial fossa and the temporal lobe is the tegmen tympani.
- **Inferior** – separating the region from the bulb of the jugular is a thin sheet of the petrous temporal bone.
- **Anterior** – the tympanic tube communicates with the pharynx.
- **Posterior** – the mastoid antrum is accessed via the aditus.

What two muscles are found in the middle ear and what is their function?

The **tensor tympani** arises from the edge of the tympanic tube and is attached to the malleus, and is supplied by the nerve to the medial pterygoid from the mandibular branch of the trigeminal nerve.

The **stapedius** is attached to the medial wall of the stapes and is supplied by the facial nerve. In Bells palsy, there is often hyperacusis due to paralysis of the stapedius muscle, which normally dampens the conduction of vibration through the ossicular chain.

What parasympathetic nerves run through the region?

The **lesser petrosal nerve** runs from the tympanic branch of the glossopharyngeal nerve to supply the parotid.

The **chorda tympani** runs from the facial nerve as it courses medial to the space to run between the two layers of the pars flaccida of the tympanic membrane. It then leaves anteriorly via the petrotympanic fissure to join the lingual branch of the mandibular division of the trigeminal nerve to supply the submandibular and sublingual salivary glands.

22   GALLBLADDER AND BILIARY TREE

What is the surface marking of the gallbladder?

- The gallbladder is situated in its fossa between the right lobe of the liver and the quadrate lobe. It is inferiorly related to the duodenum and transverse colon.
- Its surface marking is the ninth costal cartilage at the lateral edge of the rectus abdominis.
- The fundus of the gallbladder lies in the transpyloric plane of Addison at L1.

What is the arterial supply of the gallbladder?

The gallbladder is supplied by the cystic artery, most commonly a branch from the right hepatic artery. However, numerous anatomical variants exist, including an origin from the common hepatic artery. The gallbladder also draws a supply from its hepatic bed and this is evidenced clinically when cholecystitis causes thrombosis of the cystic artery.

Describe the approach steps taken in performing a laparoscopic cholecystectomy.

The patient should undergo preoperative preparation with a full history, examination and investigations, including full blood count (FBC), urea and electrolytes (U&Es), liver function tests (LFTs), amylase, clotting screen and ultrasound of the liver and gallbladder. Other relevant pathology, such as hiatus hernia and peptic ulcer disease should be excluded and an assessment of the cardiovascular and respiratory systems made. Contraindications to laparoscopic cholecystectomy should be discussed.

Then, when appropriately worked up and after informed valid consent has been obtained (including the possibility of conversion to an open procedure), and with the patient under a general anaesthetic in the supine position, the whole abdomen is prepared and draped.

A peumoperitoneum is induced using the Hassan cannulation technique (open/direct vision) just below the umbilicus and a 10-mm port is inserted. Three further incisions are made under laparoscopic vision: another 10-mm port in the subxiphisternum; and two 5-mm ports, one in the right upper quadrant and one inferiorly in the region of the right iliac fossa.

After a full laparoscopy of the abdomen has been performed, the triangle of Calot is displayed by division of the peritoneum on its anterior and posterior aspects. The cystic artery is divided between ligaclips, a cholangiogram is performed if required, and then the cystic duct is divided between ligaclips and the gallbladder removed from its bed. Haemostasis is achieved and the ports withdrawn. The fascial layer of the 10-mm ports is closed with 1 Vicryl.

23   LIVER

Describe the blood supply to the liver.

- 80% of the blood supply is derived from the portal vein.
- 20% is from the common hepatic artery, a branch of the coeliac axis, which gives off the gastroduodenal artery before branching into right and left hepatic arteries, to supply the right and left lobes respectively.

Anatomical variations in vessels is common and important. Can you give some examples in the liver?

- The right hepatic artery may branch off the superior mesenteric artery, passing posterior to the uncinate process and head of the pancreas to run on the posterior surface of the bile duct.
- The blood supply to the left lobe of the liver may be derived from the left gastric branch of the coeliac axis, with a vessel running within the lesser omentum.

How may the knowledge of the blood supply to the liver be utilised in the treatment of liver disease?

- The liver is divided into eight segments that may be segmentally removed because each is supplied by a branch of the hepatic artery, portal vein and bile duct.
- The presence of hepatic metastases, for example from a colorectal carcinoma, does not preclude resection of the primary and palliative measures, because up to 70% of the liver may be resected, with the remaining parenchyma undergoing regeneration.
- In the treatment of unresectable colorectal metastases, selective portal vein embolisation results in atrophy of the affected lobe and hypertrophy of the unaffected lobe. This is utilised when extensive resection of liver parenchyma is being considered, which would otherwise leave the patient at risk of post-resection liver failure due to a subcritical residual mass of hepatic tissue.

24   ANATOMICAL SNUFFBOX

What is the anatomical snuffbox?

The anatomical snuffbox is a triangular space in the dorsum of the wrist, bounded on the radial side by the tendons of extensor pollicis brevis and abductor pollicis longus, and on the ulnar side by the tendon of extensor pollicis longus.

The **floor** is formed by the radial styloid, scaphoid, trapezium and the base of the first metacarpal.

The **roof** is formed by the deep fascia: superficial to this lies the cephalic vein and the cutaneous branch of the radial nerve; deep to this lies the radial artery.

What is the blood supply to the scaphoid and why is it important?

The major blood supply is from the radial artery. The scaphoid is supplied by dorsal vessels just distal to the waist area, which run in a retrograde fashion proximally. Thus, a fracture of the scaphoid places the proximal pole at risk of avascular necrosis. The more proximal the fracture, the more likely it is that avascular necrosis will occur.

What other bones are at particular risk of avascular necrosis?

Femoral head: The retinacular vessels arise from the trochanteric anastomosis and ascend the femoral neck under the reflected fibres of the joint capsule to supply the femoral head. Intra-capsular fractures of the femoral neck therefore often result in avascular necrosis.

Talus: The blood supply is from an anastomosis contributed to by dorsalis pedis, the posterior tibial artery and the peroneal arteries. These vessels supply the talus through the neck and the sinus tarsi beneath. Displaced fractures of the talar neck put the talar body at risk of avascular necrosis.

25   SHOULDER

What type of joint is found in the shoulder and what contributes to its stability?

The shoulder joint is a synovial ball and socket joint between the humeral head and the glenoid. It is an intrinsically unstable joint because of the disproportionate sizes of the humeral head and glenoid. Factors that contribute to the stability of this joint are:

*   The glenoid labrum, which deepens the socket
*   The capsule, which is strengthened by the fusion of the rotator cuff muscles with it (but therefore weak inferiorly)
*   Ligaments – glenohumeral, coracohumeral and coracoacromial ligaments
*   Muscles – the rotator cuff muscles, subscapularis, supraspinatus, infraspinatus and teres minor
*   Tendons – the long head of biceps and triceps.

What are the anatomical mechanisms of shoulder dislocations?

*   **Anterior dislocation** – most common. The humeral head abducts and externally rotates out of the joint, to lie anterior to the scapula, usually subcoracoid or subclavicular. The arm is usually kept in slight abduction and externally rotated.
*   **Posterior dislocation** – the humeral head is displaced backwards by adduction and internal rotation, or occasionally by a direct blow. The arm is held in adduction and internal rotation.
*   **Inferior dislocation** (luxatio erecta) – commonly caused by hyperabduction of the humerus with the neck of the humerus levering against the acromion. The humeral head is displaced inferiorly and arm is locked in the overhead position (abduction).

Describe the surgical approaches to the shoulder.

Two common approaches are the anterior and posterior approaches.

Anterior approach: Expose the deltopectoral groove. This is marked by the cephalic vein. Ligate its branches and retract the vein. Open down the groove. Retract deltoid laterally to expose the coracoid process and its attachments. Detach the tip of the coracoid process or make a step-cut in the conjoint tendon (the musculocutaneous nerve is at risk here entering coracobrachialis), exposing subscapularis beneath. Externally rotate the shoulder to stretch subscapularis – this can be cut to enter the shoulder joint.

Posterior approach: Skin incision from the acromion going along the spine of the scapula to expose deltoid. Detach deltoid from the scapular spine and retract it laterally to reveal infraspinatus and teres minor. These can be cut to expose the joint capsule. The axillary nerve and posterior circumflex humeral artery are at risk as they pass through the quadrangular space just distal to teres minor to enter the deltoid.

26   ELBOW

What is the antecubital fossa?

The antecubital fossa is a triangular space on the anterior aspect of the elbow, bordered laterally by brachioradialis, medially by pronator teres and proximally by a line between the two epicondyles. The **floor** is formed by brachialis and the proximal end of supinator; the **roof** is formed by the deep fascia reinforced by the bicipital aponeurosis. Superficial to this lies the median cubital vein. Deep to this, the fossa contains the median nerve, brachial artery, biceps tendon, the radial nerve and its branch, the posterior interosseous nerve.

What type of joint is found in the elbow and what movements does it provide?

The elbow joint is a synovial joint of the hinge variety between the distal humerus and the proximal radius and ulna. The olecranon and the trochlear are closely congruent and provide stability. The only movements at this joint are flexion and extension. Pronation and supination of the forearm are provided by the radioulnar joints and not by the elbow joint.

What neurovascular structures are at risk in a supracondylar fracture of the humerus?

Supracondylar fractures are common in childhood, resulting from a fall on the outstretched hand. Displaced fractures are commonly accompanied by neurovascular damage as a result of impingement against the spike of the proximal fracture site. The brachial artery may be 'kinked' by the dorsally displaced distal fragment. Injury to the median nerve (especially to its anterior interosseous branch), or to the radial or ulnar nerves, is also common.

27   FLEXOR SHEATHS

What are the flexor sheaths?

The flexor tendons are invested in synovial sheaths. They have a visceral and a parietal layer and contain synovial fluid, providing nutrition and lubrication functions for the tendons. The synovial sheath is surrounded by a fibrous sheath between the metacarpal heads and the distal phalanx. It has its base on the phalanges, forming fibro-osseous tunnels for the passage of the tendons. This keeps the tendons close to the bones and joints during finger movements. The fibres are laid down in an annular, cruciate and transverse manner along the way, to form pulleys, which prevent bowstringing of the tendon during flexion. They also act as fulcrums for flexion.

How are the flexor and extensor tendons attached to the phalanges?

Flexors: The superficialis tendon enters the fibrous flexor sheath and divides into two halves. These spiral round the profundus tendon to partially decussate before inserting into the front of the middle phalanx. The profundus tendon enters the fibrous sheath, initially deep to the superficialis tendon. It then passes through the tendon to become superficial to it and continues on to insert into the base of the distal phalanx.

Extensors: The extensor expansion splits into three parts. The central part inserts into the middle phalanx while the collateral slips converge onto the base of the distal phalanx. (Note the opposite pattern of insertion to the flexor tendons.)

What is flexor tenosynovitis and why is it important?

Flexor tenosynovitis is an orthopaedic emergency. It is an infection that spreads within the flexor tendon sheath, which can lead to scarring of the tendon and sheath and tendon necrosis, resulting in loss of finger function. Clinically it is suggested by the presence of **Kanavel's signs:**

- Intense pain on attempted extension
- Flexion posturing of the finger
- Uniform swelling of the finger
- Tenderness over the tendon sheath.

Treatment is by incision and drainage, followed by irrigation of the flexor sheath for 48 hours. Very early infection may occasionally be managed initially with a trial of antibiotic therapy.

28   BONY PELVIS

What kind of joint is the sacroiliac joint?

The sacroiliac joint is a synovial joint between the auricular surfaces of the ilium and sacrum. In the upright position, the body weight tends to push the sacrum downwards and rotate it forwards on the pelvis. The angulation of the joint surfaces does not oppose this, and therefore the ligaments are very important for the stability of the sacroiliac joint. The anterior, posterior and interosseous sacroiliac ligaments reinforce the joint capsule; together with the iliolumbar ligaments, they oppose caudal displacement of the sacrum. The sacroiliac and sacrospinous ligaments are attached to the lower end of the sacrum to oppose the forward rotation of the sacrum on the pelvis.

What is the anatomical position for the pelvis?

In the anatomical position, the anterior superior iliac spine and the superior end of the symphysis pubis lie in the same vertical plane. The tip of the coccyx, the ischial spines and the upper border of the symphysis pubis also lie in the same horizontal plane.

What are the differences between the male and female pelvis?

The pelvis has evolved for its function as a major weight-bearing structure but in the female it also needs to be able to accommodate a fetus. The differences can be divided into those in the birth canal and those in the rest of the pelvis:

Differences in the birth canal:

- The male pelvic inlet is heart-shaped and the female inlet is more oval-shaped. This is due to the maximum transverse diameter being more dorsal and the sacral promontory more prominent in the male.
- The male pelvis is deeper and more conical whereas the female pelvis is shallower.
- The subpubic angle is <70° in the male, and >80° in the female.
- The ischial spines are closer together and inverted in the male.

Differences in the rest of the pelvis:

- Males are more muscular and the pelvis has more marked muscular attachment markings.
- The acetabulum is larger in the male.
- The lumbosacral joint is broader in the male.

29   RADIAL NERVE PALSY

Describe the course of the radial nerve and its surface markings.

- The radial nerve is a branch of the posterior cord of the brachial plexus.
- It exits the axilla through the triangular space bordered by the shaft of the humerus, long head of triceps and teres major.
- It then exits the posterior compartment by piercing the lateral intermuscular septum into the cubital fossa. Here it divides into its superficial branch (a sensory nerve still called the radial nerve), and its motor branch (the posterior interosseous nerve, which spirals round the proximal end of the radius between the two heads of supinator to enter and supply the extensors of the forearm).
- The radial nerve continues within the forearm under brachioradialis. It is briefly joined by the radial artery, which runs medial to it, before diving backwards to the posterior forearm to supply the skin of the dorsal wrist and hand.

Its surface marking is from where the posterior wall of the axilla meets the arm, to a point two-thirds along from the acromion to the lateral epicondyle. From here it runs to the front of the epicondyle, and continues under brachioradialis to exit its dorsal edge two-thirds of the way down the forearm. The nerve can be rolled on the tendons of the anatomical snuffbox.

The posterior interosseous nerve is marked by three fingers' breadth below the radial head as it enters supinator.

What are the neurological findings in radial nerve palsy?

Injuries to the radial nerve principally lead to a motor deficit, but overlap with the median and ulnar nerves results in a small area of sensory loss over the first dorsal web space. Classically, radial nerve palsy results in a 'wrist drop' deformity due to loss of forearm extensor function. There will also be weakness in metacarpophalangeal joint extension (though the lumbricals can still extend the interphalangeal joints through their insertion into the extensor sheath). In addition, lesions in the axilla result in loss of elbow extension (but not in lesions below the axilla because the supply to the long head comes off high up).

Where are the common sites of injury to the radial nerve?

- **Axilla** – 'crutch palsy' or 'Saturday night palsy'
- **Humeral shaft** – humeral shaft fractures (especially the middle third), humeral shaft plating

- **Proximal radius** – approaches to the radial head (the posterior interosseous nerve)
- **Posterior interosseous nerve** – entrapment of the posterior interosseous nerve as it passes between the two heads of supinator.

30   ULNAR NERVE PALSY

Describe the course of the ulnar nerve and its surface markings.

• The ulnar nerve is the largest branch of the medial cord of the brachial plexus.

• It runs down the arm between the axillary nerve and vein before piercing the medial intermuscular septum at the lower third of the arm to enter the posterior compartment. Here it grooves the posterior surface of the medial epicondyle.

• From here it passes between the two heads of flexor carpi ulnaris to enter the forearm; it is joined on its lateral side by the ulnar artery. They continue together down the forearm between flexor carpi ulnaris and flexor digitorum profundus.

• At the wrist, the nerve emerges lateral to the tendon of flexor carpi ulnaris to run superficial to the flexor retinaculum in 'Guyon's canal' to enter the hand.

Surface markings: In the arm, the ulnar nerve runs from a point two-thirds of the way along the anterior axillary fold to the medial epicondyle. It is palpable on the groove on the posterior surface of the medial epicondyle. In the forearm, it lies along a line running from the medial epicondyle of the humerus to the radial side of the pisiform.

What are the neurological findings in ulnar nerve palsy?

Classically, ulnar nerve palsy presents with a **claw hand**. Here, the metacarpophalangeal joints are hyperextended and the interphalangeal joints are flexed due to loss of intrinsic muscle function in the hand. The defect is more pronounced in the ring and little fingers because the first two lumbricals are supplied by the median nerve. Clawing is more severe in distal lesions (**the ulnar paradox**) because clawing requires the action of flexor digitorum profundus. The ulnar half of this muscle is supplied by the ulnar nerve, and when it is paralysed by a high ulnar nerve lesion, the clawing is less severe.

In long-standing lesions, wasting of the small muscles of the hand results in guttering between the metacarpals, especially between the first and second metacarpals (first dorsal interosseous wasting). There is sensory loss over the ulnar one and a half digits, although this is variable due to overlapping innervation.

Where are the common sites of injury to the ulnar nerve?

Most commonly injured at the elbow (due to elbow fractures) or the wrist (where the nerve lies superficially; usually due to lacerations).

Sites of entrapment:

- Cubital tunnel (commonly between the two heads of flexor carpi ulnaris)
- Guyon's canal.

4

OPERATIVE SURGERY

1   FASCIOTOMY

Name the compartments of the lower leg and what is found within them.

Anterior (extensor compartment):

- Muscles – tibialis anterior, extensor hallucis longus, extensor digitorum longus and peroneus tertius
- Nerve – deep peroneal nerve
- Vessels – anterior tibial artery.

Lateral (peroneal):

- Muscles – peroneus longus and brevis
- Nerve – superficial peroneal nerve
- Vessels – peroneal artery and small saphenous vein.

Supericial and deep posterior (flexor):

- Superficial muscles – gastrocnemius, plantaris and soleus, with underlying deep transverse fascia separating them from deep muscles
- Deep muscles – popliteus, flexor digitorum longus, flexor hallucis longus, tibialis posterior
- Nerve – tibial division of the sciatic nerve
- Vessels – posterior tibial artery and its peroneal branch.

When would you suspect a compartment syndrome?

- Pain out of proportion to the injury
- Pain on passive stretching of the involved compartment
- Paralysis and paraesthesia are late signs.

How would you treat compartment syndrome?

This is a surgical emergency.

- Split plasters/bandages (if present) down to skin or take them off completely and perform urgent fasciotomy of all involved compartments.
- Double incision technique with perifibular fasciotomy.
- Decompress superficial and deep posterior compartment through medial longitudinal incision placed 1–2 cm posterior to medial border of the tibia, keeping anterior to posterior tibial artery to avoid injury to perforating vessels that supply local fasciocutaneous flaps.
- Decompress anterior and lateral compartments through longitudinal incision 2 cm lateral to anterior tibial border.

2   CERVICAL LYMPH NODE BIOPSY

How would you carry out a cervical lymph node biopsy?

- Fully inform the patient and obtain consent.
- Perform under general anaesthetic.
- Place the patient in a supine position, with sandbags under their shoulders to improve surgical exposure.
- Place the incision over the node, taking care to avoid damage to important anatomical structures, such as nerves or major vessels (eg the cervical branch of the facial nerve, running below the border of the mandible).
- Make an incision through the skin, subcutaneous fat and fascia, down to the lymph node; dissect to free the lymph node with careful haemostasis and ligation of lymph vessels.
- Obtain a fresh specimen for immunohistochemical staining if lymphoma is suspected.
- Specimen may be fixed in 10% formalin and sent to the pathology laboratory.
- If tuberculosis is suspected, obtain a fresh specimen for acid alcohol-fast staining.
- Send pus to microbiology for microscopy, culture and sensitivity.
- Close in layers with absorbable sutures.
- Local anaesthetic infiltration for postoperative analgesia.

What would you do if you find the lymph node is intramuscular or adherent to the internal jugular vein?

- Carefully dissect in line with muscle fibres.
- If densely adherent to a major structure, take a wedge excision biopsy of the superficial part of the lymph node.
- Keep deep part undisturbed to allow histological diagnosis and to avoid injury to the structure.

What would you do if the patient had ear, nose and throat (ENT) symptoms?

- Preoperative ENT assessment to exclude tumour is required.
- Cancel the biopsy and refer the patient to ENT.
- Laryngeal tumours require a laryngectomy and block dissection of the cervical lymph nodes, and excision biopsy of a metastatic cervical lymph node could influence long-term prognosis.

3   CHEST DRAIN

What are the indications for a chest drain?

Pneumothorax:

- Trauma
- Bullae rupture in chronic obstructive pulmonary disease
- Iatrogenic
- Spontaneous
- Tension.

Haemothorax:

- Trauma
- Postoperative.

Chylothorax:

- Postoperative
- Cannulation of left subclavian vein complicated by injury to thoracic duct.

Massive effusion.

Empyema.

Prophylactic – after cardiothoracic, oesophageal or spinal surgery.

How do you insert a chest drain?

- Explain procedure (verbal consent).
- Infiltrate with local anaesthesia and prepare skin with Betadine® (povidone-iodine).
- Landmarks – fifth intercostal space, mid-axillary line, superior to rib.
- Stab skin incision.
- Blunt dissection through intercostal muscles and pleura using Roberts clamp.
- Insert drain over curved Roberts clamp.

What are the structures to be avoided?

- Neurovascular structures underneath each rib
- Long thoracic nerve (of Bell) lying behind the mid-axillary line – injury causes weakness of serratus anterior, leading to winging of scapula.

4   CARPAL TUNNEL DECOMPRESSION

How would you perform carpal tunnel decompression?

- Fully inform the patient and obtain consent.
- Local anaesthetic and tourniquet.
- Incision in line with third web space distal to the distal wrist crease (painful scar if incised through the crease).
- Proximal to the line of first web space (thenar eminence).
- Ensure skin incision is perpendicular to the skin.
- Protect the nerve with a Macdonald's dissector.
- Check flexor retinaculum is fully released (proximal and distal).

What are the contents and bony attachments of the carpal tunnel?

Contents:

- Flexor digitorum superficialis
- Flexor digitorum profundus
- Flexor pollicis longus
- Median nerve
- Flexor carpi radialis (splits ligament).

Attachments:

- Pisiform, hook of hamate (ulnar)
- Tubercle of scaphoid, ridge of trapezium (radial).

What other structures are at risk during this procedure?

- Palmaris longus
- Palmar cutaneous branch of the median nerve
- Superficial branch of the radial artery
- Ulnar artery and nerve
- Recurrent motor branch of the median nerve.
- Palmar arch (superficial and deep).

5   TRACHEOSTOMY

What are the indications for tracheostomy?

- Acute airway compromise despite attempts to secure a definitive non-surgical airway
- Long-term ventilation
- For management of airway with laryngeal pathology
- Lung toilet
- To reduce the work of breathing by reducing dead space for breathing.

How do you perform an elective tracheostomy?

- Fully inform the patient and obtain consent.
- Secure an established airway.
- Make a horizontal incision midway between the thyroid notch and the sternal notch.
- Identify strap muscles and dissect them in the midline.
- Identify the cricoid cartilage, thyroid and trachea (inferiorly).
- Divide and ligate the thyroid isthmus.
- Identify the first to fourth tracheal rings.
- Check the tracheostomy tube (check cuff, connections and inner tube); have suction and tracheal dilators available.
- Inform the anaesthetist of readiness to perform tracheostomy.
- Anaesthetist to loosen endotracheal tube.
- Excise ring – two-thirds anterior cartilage window.
- Insert tracheostomy.
- Suction of airway.
- Close wound loosely.
- Suture tracheostomy tube in situ.
- Also tie tube around the neck snugly.
- Tracheostomy-competent nursing staff are essential.
- Keep tracheal dilators by the bedside with replacement tube.

What are the complications of tracheostomy?

Intraoperative complications:

- Injury to surrounding structures – larynx, subglottis and cricoid cartilage, oesophagus, subclavian artery and brachiocephalic vein, recurrent laryngeal nerves, thyroid gland
- Pneumothorax
- Injury to trachea – excessive tracheal stoma, injury to trachealis
- Haemorrhage.

Postoperative complications:

- **Early:**
  - general – bleeding, infection, wound dehiscence
  - specific – injury to surrounding structures, veins and arteries of the neck, difficulty with swallowing and speech, accidental decannulation
- **Late:**
  - neck scar, tracheal tethering to the skin (noticeable on swallowing), laryngeal and subglottic stenosis (with long-term intubation).

6   SKIN BIOPSY

What types of biopsies are you aware of?

Needle biopsy:

- Fine-needle aspiration ± guidance, eg pancreas or breast
- Trucut needle, eg kidney, breast.

Surgical biopsy:

- Excision for small lesions, eg of skin, lymph nodes when architecture is important, polyps (including base)
- Incisional if too large for excision, representative of full lesion depth including margin and adjacent normal tissue.

How do you perform a skin lesion biopsy?

- Fully inform the patient and obtain consent; local anaesthetic, clean and drape the area.
- Mask the chosen excision margin, with an ellipse with length 3× width.
- Cut perpendicular to the skin thoughout full thickness, keeping tension on skin with hooks.
- Dissect out the full thickness of the lesion, using diathermy for haemostasis.
- Remove lesion, tag if needed and send in correctly labelled pot in appropriate fluid (or dry).
- Check haemostasis.
- Close wound without tension.

What are the complications of a skin biopsy?

Immediate complications:

- Anaesthetic complications
- Haemorrhage
- Damage to adjacent structures.

Early complications:

- Wound infection/breakdown.

Late complications:

- Incomplete excision
- Seeding
- Recurrence
- Metastatic spread after incomplete resection
- False-negative biopsy result
- Keloid and hypertrophic scarring.

7 LAPAROTOMY INCISIONS

What are the important considerations when planning an abdominal incision?

- Adequate access to underlying tissues or structures
- Position (over lesion, away from bony prominences)
- Parallel to Langer's lines (along natural lines of tension – heal better)
- Parallel to important structures
- Cosmesis (inside natural creases, Pfannenstiel for pelvic surgery)
- Ensure incision is perpendicular to skin.

What abdominal incisions are you aware of and what are their advantages and disadvantages?

Transverse:

- Good access in children, secure healing, fewer chest problems
- Inadequate in adults, difficult to extend, longer to open and close, more blood loss, especially if cutting muscle.

Midline:

- Good access, easy to extend, quick to open and close, less blood loss
- More painful, less cosmetic than transverse.

Paramedian:

- Effective closure without strong sutures, low hernia rate
- Takes longer to close.

Roof top: good access for oesophagus, stomach, liver and pancreatic surgery.

Kocker: good access for gallbladder surgery.

How do you close a laparotomy wound?

- Midline laparotomy and transverse wounds may be closed by 'mass closure'.
- Paramedian incisions need musculo-aponeurotic closure in layers.
- Mass closure has lower incidence of dehiscence but same incisional hernia rate.
  - Over-and-over continuous closure with suture length 4× wound length (Jenkins 1976).
  - Sutures placed 1 cm apart with 1-cm bites.
  - Suture material – 1 nylon or 1 PDS, loop or non-looped.

8 TESTICULAR TORSION

How would you prepare an 18-year-old man for exploration of the testis for possible testicular torsion?

- Full history and examination
- Recognition of surgical emergency (irreversible damage in <4 hours)
- Identify anaesthetic risks
- Informed consent (including possibility of orchidectomy and contralateral testis exploration).

What are the principles of the procedure?

Incisions:

- Transverse (bilateral)
- Midline raphe incision.

Layers:

- Skin
- Dartos (Colles', Scarpa's) fascia
- External spermatic fascia (external oblique)
- Cremasteric fascia (internal oblique)
- Internal spermatic fascia (transversalis)
- Parietal tunica vaginalis
- Testis.

Procedure:

- Inspection of colour, cord, fluid, epididymis, testicular and epididymal appendages, palpation of testis
- De-tort the testis, warm gauze, observation
- Fixation of the testis.

How do you fix the testicle if it is viable?

- Three-point fixation with non-absorbable prolene (eg 4/0), **or** formation of 'Dartos pouch'
- Fixation to scrotal wall, or fixation of testis to parietal tunica vaginalis alone (no fixation required in Dartos pouch method)
- Contralateral exploration and fixation of testis ('bell clapper' deformity).

9   SUPRAPUBIC CATHETERISATION

What methods of suprapubic catheterisation are available?

- Adacath (Bard)
- Banano catheter
- Needle drainage
- Open technique.

How would you perform a suprapubic catheterisation, and what precautions would you take?

- History and examination to identify the presence of a distended bladder
- Verbal consent
- Check for coagulation disorder
- Antibiotic prophylaxis
- Prepare and drape (patient supine)
- Anaesthetise skin and subcutaneous tissues
- Introduce a needle 2 cm above symphysis pubis, aiming slightly caudally
- Aspirate urine
- Make a 1-cm incision over the needle mark
- Place Adacath into the bladder
- Remove obturator
- Introduce catheter
- 'Peel' off Adacath.

What are the main complications of performing suprapubic catheterisation?

Early complications:

- Failure
- Infection
- Bleeding
- Perforation of bowel segment
- Displacement.

Late complications:

- Blockage
- Encrustation
- Stones
- Contracted bladder
- Urinary tract infection
- Inflammatory changes – transitional cell carcinoma.

10   FEMORAL EMBOLECTOMY

Describe the anatomy of the femoral triangle.

Base – inguinal ligament.
Lateral border – sartorius.
Medial border – adductor longus.

Contents:

- Femoral canal (node of Cloquet)
- Femoral vein
- Femoral artery
- Femoral nerve
- Long saphenous vein.

What are the classic symptoms and signs of acute limb ischaemia?

Sudden onset of:

- Pain
- Pallor
- Pulselessness
- Paraesthesia
- Paralysis
- Perishing cold (poikilothermia).

What are the principles of a femoral embolectomy?

- The patient is fully heparinised.
- The anaesthetic can be general or local.
- The involved artery is exposed and proximal and distal control is achieved.
- A suitable size of Fogarty catheter is selected (size 3 for femoral); the balloon is tested with saline.
- Arteriotomy is performed (ideally a transverse arteriotomy as it reduces the risk of stenosis on closure).
- The uninflated catheter is passed beyond the site of the clot and pulled back – the aim is to keep the balloon apposed to the arterial wall by gently inflating and deflating as the calibre of the artery changes.
- The catheter is pulled out through the arteriotomy and the embolus is recovered.
- This procedure is performed proximally and distally.
- The proximal and distal artery are then flushed with heparinised saline.
- The arteriotomy is closed with 4/0 prolene sutures.

11   CHRONIC LIMB ISCHAEMIA

What is the definition of 'rest pain'?

Pain in the forefoot at rest, especially at night, relieved by dependency and associated with an absolute ankle pressure of <50 mmHg.

What are the principles of reconstructive arterial surgery?

Indications:

- Critical ischaemia (ie rest pain, tissue loss or gangrene)
- Short-distance claudication (controversial).

Principles of bypass surgery:

- The aim is to achieve straight-line arterial flow to the foot.
- Expose the inflow and outflow arteries.
- Gain adequate proximal and distal control.
- Give 5000 U unfractionated heparin prior to the application of arterial clamps.
- Make a proximal and distal anastomosis using a suitable conduit.
- Check flow in graft using hand-held Doppler.
- Assess the foot clinically for improved capillary refill, sweating (or even a palpable pulse!)

What conduits can be used and what techniques can be used to improve the long-term patency of distal bypass grafts?

Conduits:

- Autologous – vein (long saphenous vein, short saphenous vein, cephalic vein, human umbilical vein)
- Artificial – polytetrafluoroethylene (PTFE), Dacron.

Techniques to improve long-term patency:

- Use vein bypass wherever possible.
- If a prosthetic graft is used:
  - Taylor patch
  - Miller cuff
  - St Mary's boot.
- Graft surveillance.
- Antiplatelet therapy.
- Cessation of smoking.

12   BELOW-KNEE AMPUTATION

What are the indications for amputation?

The three 'D's.

Dead:

- Acute ischaemia
- Unreconstructable critical ischaemia.

Dangerous:

- Crush injury
- Gas gangrene
- Necrotising fasciitis
- Tumour.

Damn nuisance:

- Useless, insensate limb.

What are the complications associated with a below-knee amputation?

Immediate complications:

- Bleeding.

Early complications:

- Haematoma
- Wound infection
- Wound dehiscence
- Skin necrosis
- Phantom limb pain
- Oedema
- Ischaemia.

Late complications:

- Ulceration
- Neuroma.

What are the contraindications to a below-knee amputation?

- Joint contractures affecting the knee or hip
- Severe osteoarthritis of the knee
- Spasticity or paralysis of the lower leg
- Sensory neuropathy affecting the skin of a future stump
- Infection of the lower leg requiring a higher amputation
- Ischaemia of the lower leg requiring a higher amputation.

13   SURGICAL APPROACHES TO THE HIP

Describe the hip joint.

- Synovial ball and socket joint lined by hyaline articular cartilage
- Capsule – lined by synovial membrane, attached anteriorly to intertrochanteric line and posteriorly halfway along femoral neck
- Socket deepened by acetabular labrum (triangular in section) – acetabulum is horseshoe-shaped, with central pad of fat (Haversian pad) and inferior margin marked by transverse acetabular ligament
- Femoral head is two-thirds of a sphere, with fovea capitis where ligamentum teres attaches
- Ligaments:
  - iliofemoral (Y-shaped ligament, ligament of Bigalow) – attached to lower half of anterior inferior iliac spine, its base to the intertrochanteric line; limits hip extension to 20°
  - ischiofemoral – lies posteriorly and is weakest, blending with zona orbicularis of capsule
  - pubofemoral – anterior and is attached to superior ramus and obturator crest of pubic bone, passing distally deep to iliofemoral ligament and blending with capsule
- Movements – flexion/extension/abduction/adduction/rotation.

What different approaches to the hip joint are you aware of?

Medial – between gracilis and adductor longus, and then between adductor magnus and brevis.

Anterior – between tensor fascia lata (superior gluteal nerve) and sartorius (femoral nerve); then rectus femoris (femoral nerve) and gluteus medius (superior gluteal nerve).

Anterolateral – between gluteus medius and tensor fascia lata.

Lateral – through common gluteus medius insertion and vastus lateralis origin.

Posterior – through deep fascia and gluteus maximus. Note piriformis, superior gemellus, obturator internus and inferior gemellus and divide these short external rotators at their insertion.

What nerves may be damaged during hip surgery?

Medial approach:

- Posterior branch of obturator nerve
- Neurovascular bundle of gracilis.

Anterior approach – lateral femoral cutaneous nerve of thigh.
Anterolateral approach – inferior branch of superior gluteal nerve.
Lateral approach – superior gluteal nerve.
Posterior approach – sciatic nerve.

14   THYROIDECTOMY

What is the blood supply of the thyroid gland?

Arterial supply:

- Superior thyroid artery from the external carotid artery
- Inferior thyroid artery from the subclavian artery, via the thyrocervical trunk
- Midline thyroid ima artery from the aortic arch in approximately 10% of people.

Venous drainage is via three paired veins:

- Superior thyroid vein – facial or internal jugular vein
- Middle thyroid vein – internal jugular vein
- Inferior thyroid vein – brachiocephalic vein.

What are the potential risks of a thyroidectomy?

Major risks:

- Injury to recurrent laryngeal nerve, with hoarseness
- Bleeding, associated oedema and tracheal compression with stridor
- Hypocalcaemia due to parathyroid gland damage.

Minor risks:

- Scar (hypertropohic/keloid)
- Wound infection
- Pain.

Can you describe how you would perform a thyroid lobectomy?

- Fully inform the patient and obtain consent; position with shoulder roll and head ring.
- Make a collar incision two fingers' breadth above the sternal notch.
- Elevate the flap in subplatysma plane to the level of the superior border of the thyroid cartilage, superficial to the anterior jugular veins.
- Dissect in the midline to retract the strap muscles.
- Ligate the middle thyroid vein.
- Dissect the superior pole, ligate and divide superior pedicle, double-tie and transfixation ligation.
- Mobilise the inferior pole.
- Identify the recurrent laryngeal nerve, using the inferior thyroid artery as the best landmark – trachea and carotid also helpful. (Remember that the nerve can be superficial or deep or between the branches of the inferior thyroid artery.)
- Ligate the inferior thyroid artery, ideally medially in order to preserve the parathyroid gland blood supply.

- Follow the recurrent laryngeal nerve until it enters under cricopharyngeus.
- Remove the gland.
- Ensure haemostasis.
- Insert two large drains.
- Close strap muscles over the trachea (to prevent tracheal tethering to skin).
- Close the wound.

15   APPENDICECTOMY

How would you prepare a patient for an appendicectomy?

- Full history and examination
- Prepare patient for theatre
- Informed consent
- General anaesthesia; supine position
- Clean and prepare the whole abdomen (in case further procedures are deemed necessary)
- Intravenous antibiotics given at induction (must include anaerobic cover, ie metronidazole; most common combination is cefuroxime and metronidazole).

Can you describe how you would gain access to the peritoneal cavity when planning an appendicectomy, and what structures would you consider?

- Make a Lanz incision (runs along Langer's lines, 1–2 cm medial to the anterior superior iliac spine) over McBurney's point.
- Dissect through the subcutaneous fat and fascia, down to the external oblique aponeurosis.
- Make an incision through the aponeurosis, parallel to the wound incision.
- Split the muscle fibres of the external oblique, the internal oblique and transversus abdominis.
- Identify and open the peritoneum.

What are the operative steps once the peritoneum has been opened?

- Take a swab for microbiology of any peritoneal fluid (for culture).
- Inspect the caecum and small bowel for other pathology (eg Meckel's diverticulum, caecal tumours) and the ovaries and Fallopian tubes in order to exclude pelvic inflammation, ectopic pregnancy or ovarian cysts.
- Identify the taeniae coli on the caecum and follow them down to the appendix.
- Clip and divide the vessels on the mesoappendix.
- Apply a Dunhill forceps to the base of the appendix.
- Apply a surgical tie to the base and divide the base.
- Purse-string suture to the caecum to bury the appendix stump (optional step – not necessary).
- Ask for new instruments.
- Peritoneal lavage using normal saline.
- Close in layers, using absorbable sutures (eg Vicryl).
- Perform a Betadine® wound lavage to reduce the risk of wound infection.

16   LAPAROTOMY FOR OBSTRUCTION

How would you prepare and perform a laparotomy for obstruction?

- Adequately resuscitated patient
- Appropriate analgesia
- Nasogastric tube and urinary catheter
- General anaesthesia
- Position supine on table (Lloyd Davis if access to pelvis is thought necessary)
- Long midline incision, cutting through:
  - skin
  - fat
  - linea alba.

How would you identify the cause of obstruction once inside the abdomen?

Follow the dilated loops of bowel distally until the area of obstruction is reached. There will be some loops of collapsed bowel distal to it.

How would you proceed?

- Deal with the cause of the obstruction (eg hernia, adhesion or tumour).
- Free the obstructed loop.
- Assess the viability of the obstructed segment of bowel.
- Non-viable bowel should be excised (as demonstrated by poor blood supply, absence of peristalsis, no pulsation of mesenteric vessels, loss of sheen on the surface of the bowel).
- A primary bowel anastomosis may be safely performed in the absence of faecal contamination in a haemodynamically stable patient.
- Anastomosis can be performed if there is purulent contamination, but only by an experienced surgical and anaesthetic team.
- A proximal diverting loop stoma should be considered if a primary large-bowel anastomosis is performed.

17   INGUINAL HERNIAS

What types of inguinal hernia are you aware of?

- Indirect
- Direct
- Combined ('pantaloon' hernia).

How would you differentiate between a direct and an indirect inguinal hernia?

Clinically:

Put a finger over the midpoint of the inguinal canal (over the deep ring):

- If the swelling is controlled, then it is an indirect hernia.
- If the hernia bulges medial to finger (ie through the muscle wall of the inguinal canal), then it is a direct hernia.

At surgery:

Relationship to inferior epigastric artery:

- Direct hernial sac lies medial to the artery.
- Indirect hernial sac lies lateral to the artery.

How would you repair an indirect inguinal hernia?

- Obtain informed consent.
- Place the patient in the supine position, with adequate skin preparation.
- Give a single dose of antibiotics (eg cefuroxime given at induction).
- Make a transverse skin incision in the groin crease overlying the hernia, through subcutaneous fat and Scarpa's fascia to the external oblique aponeurosis.
- Expose the superficial ring and open the inguinal canal to expose the spermatic cord and its contents.
- Carefully examine the cord to identify the presence of a hernial sac.
- Dissect the hernial sac off the spermatic cord, taking care with the contents of the cord (including the vessels and the vas).
- The cremasteric vessels may need to be ligated and divided to gain access and to achieve full haemostasis.
- Open the sac to identify any bowel or omentum contents within it.
- Transfix and excise the sac.
- Repair and reinforce the weakened posterior wall of the inguinal canal using a mesh (eg Prolene) using the Lichtenstein technique.

- Close the wound in layers using absorbable sutures (eg Vicryl).
- Infiltrate the wound with local anaesthetic.

18   BURR HOLE

When would you contemplate attempting an emergency burr hole?

Only in exceptional circumstances, and after having received the appropriate training – **neurosurgical advice is essential** when performing an emergency burr hole. This procedure might be considered in the following circumstances:

- Rapidly deteriorating neurological status when transfer to a neurosurgical unit is not possible or will create a long delay
- Evidence of ipsilateral mass effect, ie hemiparesis, dilated pupil
- Failure of non-surgical measures (ie sedation and paralysis (accompanied by mechanical ventilation), short-term hypocapnia and mannitol diuretic).

Where can you make a burr hole?

Temporal burr hole – 2 cm anterior and 4 cm superior to the external auditory meatus.

Frontal burr hole – mid-pupillary line and 2 cm posterior to the coronal suture.

Parietal burr hole – over the convexity of the parietal eminence.

How would you perform an emergency burr hole operation?

Consent – proceed with the confidence that the operation is being performed to immediately save life; complete NHS Consent Form 4 in retrospect and explain to the family.

Anaesthetic – unlikely to influence a comatose patient, but the patient needs an endotracheal tube and intermittent positive-pressure ventilation, plus sedation and paralysis for control of intracranial pressure; administer lidocaine and adrenaline locally after prepping if time permits.

Position – supine, with head in a neutral position on a head ring and 20°–30° head-up postion.

Preparation – shave if time permits.

Incision – make a 4-cm linear incision over the maximum depth of the haematoma as shown on computed tomography. (Remember that this may modify the classic exploratory burr hole sites as described above.)

Exposure – incise all the way down to bone, retract with mastoid self-retractor forceps, and scrape away pericranium with a periosteal elevator.

Drilling – ensure perforator drill bit is attached to the Hudson brace. Position yourself comfortably, holding the twist with one hand and the top of the brace with the other. Place drill at a right angle to the skull surface, lean in to provide force, and drill. Continue until inner cortex is just breached. If correctly positioned for an extradural haematoma, clot will ooze out; otherwise, dura can be seen. Change to a burr drill bit. The conical hole can now be enlarged to a cylindrical burr hole. Apply suction to the surface of the burr hole to evacuate the clot. **Do not pass it into the cranial cavity blind.**

Closure – approximate the wound edges and apply skin clips or loose skin sutures and dressing. **By not closing the galea aponeurosis layer, further clot can ooze out if it re-accumulates.**

Postoperatively – await transfer to the neurosurgical unit for definitive craniotomy. Continue close monitoring.

19 LUMBAR PUNCTURE

At what level does the spinal cord terminate in the adult?

The level of the lower border of the first lumbar vertebra (L1).

Which surface landmark could you use to ensure safe passage of the needle and what anatomical structures does the needle pass through to enter the subarachnoid space?

A line joining the iliac crests passes through the fourth lumbar vertebra, so the intervertebral space above or below the landmark can be used with safety.

The anatomical structures passed through are:

- Skin
- Superficial fascia
- Supraspinous ligament
- Interspinous ligament
- Ligamentum flavum
- Areolar tissue (containing internal vertebral venous plexus in the epidural space)
- Dura mater
- Arachnoid mater.

Can you name a common complication of lumbar puncture and when is the procedure contraindicated?

A common complication is post-lumbar puncture headache (approximately 30% incidence).

Contraindications to lumbar puncture include:

- Raised intracranial pressure
- Bleeding diathesis
- Infection at the site of needle insertion
- Cardiorespiratory compromise.

20   CENTRAL LINE INSERTION

What is the Seldinger technique and which vessels are commonly used for central venous access?

Seldinger technique:

- The technique involves inserting a hollow metal needle into the vein.
- A flexible guide wire is threaded through the needle that is then removed.
- A tapered dilator and plastic catheter is inserted over the guide wire and advanced into the vein.
- The guidewire and dilator are removed and the cannula secured.

Vessels used for central access:

- Internal jugular vein
- Subclavian vein
- Femoral vein.

How would you perform internal jugular and subclavian vein cannulations?

For both methods, the skin is prepared and locally anaesthetised and the area draped. The Seldinger technique is employed for cannulation.

Internal jugular cannulation:

- Place the patient in the supine position, tilted at least 15° head down, with the head turned away from the side of cannulation.
- Introduce the needle into the centre of the triangle formed by the two lower heads of sternocleidomastoid and the clavicle.
- Direct the needle inferiorly, parallel to the sagittal plane and at 30° to the skin.

Subclavian vein cannulation:

- Infraclavicular approach.
- Place the patient in the supine position, at least 15° head down, with the head turned away from the side of cannulation.
- Introduce the needle 2 cm below the midpoint of the clavicle.
- Direct the needle deep to the clavicle, pointing to the jugular notch.

After these procedures, correct positioning is confirmed and pneumothorax and haemothorax are excluded with a chest X-ray.

21   FEMORAL HERNIA

What are the boundaries of the femoral canal?

Anterior border – inguinal ligament.
Posterior border – pectineal ligament.
Medial border – lacunar ligament.
Lateral border – femoral vein.

What approaches do you know for a femoral hernia repair?

Three classic approaches to the femoral canal have been described:

- Low (Lockwood)
- Transinguinal (Lotheissen)
- High (McEvedy).

Irrespective of which approach is used, the following principles apply:

- Dissection of the sac
- Reduction/inspection of the contents
- Ligation of the sac
- Repair includes an approximation of the inguinal and pectineal ligaments; alternatively, mesh plugs can be used.

Which surgical approach would you use for a strangulated hernia and can you describe the layers you would need to dissect through?

For a strangulated femoral hernia, a high approach should be used as bowel resection may be necessary. It is performed via an oblique incision above the pubic tubercle.

The layers are:

- Skin
- Subcutaneous tissue
- Rectus sheath
- Rectus abdominis
- Transversalis fascia (note that there is no posterior leaf of rectus sheath as this is below the arcuate line)
- Peritoneum.

22   CAROTID ENDARTERECTOMY

Which preoperative imaging modalities may be used to establish the diagnosis of carotid stenosis?

- Colour duplex ultrasound
- Digital subtraction angiography.

At what level does the common carotid artery bifurcate and what nerves can be injured during surgery in this area?

The common carotid artery bifurcates at the level of the upper border of the thyroid cartilage (at vertebral level C4).

Nerves that can be damaged during carotid artery surgery:

- Vagus nerve
- Hypoglossal nerve
- Ansa cervicalis
- Cervical sympathetic chain
- External laryngeal nerve.

What are the indications for carotid endarterectomy and are you aware of any clinical trials which have looked at perioperative outcome events and risk–benefit analysis for carotid endarterectomy?

Indications for surgery:

- Symptomatic stenoses not controlled on medical therapy, ie resulting in unilateral transient ischaemic attacks (TIAs) or amaurosis fugax
- High-grade stenoses (>70%) ± neurological deficit.

North American Symptomatic Carotid Endarterectomy Trial (NASCET):

- In 1415 patients there were 92 perioperative outcome events.
- Overall rate of perioperative stroke and death was 6.5%.
- The rate of permanently disabling stroke and death was only 2.0%.
- Other surgical complications were rarely clinically important.
- Conclusion is that carotid endarterectomy is a durable procedure.

European Carotid Surgery Trial (ECST):

- Multicentre trial of patients with symptomatic carotid stenosis.
- A total of 2518 patients were randomised over 10 years.
- Patients with 'mild' stenosis (<30% stenosed): any 3-year benefits of surgery were small and outweighed by its early risks.

- Patients with 'moderate' stenosis (30%–69% stenosed): balance of surgical risk and eventual benefit remains uncertain.
- Patients with 'severe' stenosis (70%–99% stenosed): risks of surgery were significantly outweighed by the later benefits, ie a sixfold reduction in risk of ipsilateral stroke in surgery-allocated patients during the following 3 years.

23 SUBMANDIBULAR GLAND SURGERY

Where is the submandibular gland found?

The submandibular gland lies in the digastric triangle below the mandible. The **borders of the digastric triangle** are:

- **Anterior** – anterior belly of digastric
- **Posterior** – posterior belly of digastric
- **Superior** – lower border of mandible
- **Floor** – mylohyoid.

Most of the gland is superficial to the mylohyoid muscle but a small part lies deep to the mylohyoid, having passed around the posterior free border.

Can you describe the morphology and anatomical relations of the submandibular gland?

- It has a large superficial and a small deep lobe which connect with each other around the posterior border of mylohyoid.
- The superficial lobe lies at the angle of the jaw, wedged between the mandible and mylohyoid.
- Posteriorly, it comes into contact with the parotid gland.
- Superficially, it is covered by platysma and by its capsule of deep fascia. It is crossed by the cervical branch of the facial nerve and by the facial vein.
- Its deep aspect lies against the mylohyoid for the most part, but posteriorly the gland rests against hyoglossus (where it is in contact with the lingual and hypoglossal nerves).
- The facial artery approaches the gland from behind and then arches over its superior aspect.
- The submandibular duct (Wharton's duct) arises from the deep part of the gland and runs forwards to open at the side of the frenulum.

What are the potentially important complications of submandibular gland surgery and what anatomical structures may be damaged inadvertently?

- Nerve injury:
  - mandibular branch of the facial nerve – so any incision must be placed more than 2.5 cm below the angle of the jaw
  - hypoglossal nerve – lies between the deep part of the gland and hyoglossus
  - lingual nerve – lies between the deep part of the gland and hyoglossus
- Infection
- Bleeding
- Submandibular fistula (very uncommon).

24   REDUCTION OF COLLES' FRACTURE

A 70-year-old lady with osteoporosis presents with a Colles' fracture of her right wrist after falling on ice. Describe the deformity you would expect to see.

The deformity of the wrist is described as being like a 'dinner fork' and comprises the following displacements of the distal fragment:

- Impaction
- Dorsal angulation and displacement
- Radial angulation and displacement.

Describe how you would perform the reduction.

- Obtain fully informed, appropriate consent.
- Perform a haematoma block with a mixture of plain lidocaine and bupivacaine under aseptic conditions.
- With the stockinette, wool and plaster measured and cut, a reduction is obtained after traction by first exaggerating the dorsal angulation before pulling the distal fragment taut on the intact dorsal periosteum, to lever the fragment into a reduced position.
- The wrist should be held in the position of palmar flexion with a small amount of ulnar deviation in a plaster of Paris backslab, with three-point pressure applied until dry.
- The normal orientation of the distal radius is 5° of palmar angulation and 20° of ulnar deviation – this orientation should be borne in mind when reviewing the post-reduction X-rays to ascertain whether the reduction is satisfactory.

What are the late complications of this fracture that may require operative intervention?

- Malunion – corrective osteotomy
- Complex regional pain syndrome – sympathectomy in severe cases
- Carpal tunnel syndrome – release of the transverse carpal ligament
- Rupture of extensor pollicis longus – extensor indicis transfer.

25 HIP ARTHROPLASTY

What forms of hip arthroplasty do you know of?

- Total arthroplasty or hemiarthroplasty
- Cemented or uncemented
- Various bearing surfaces:
  - metal on metal
  - metal on polyethylene
  - ceramic on polyethylene
  - ceramic on ceramic.

What nerve is closely related to the posterior rim of the acetabulum and therefore at risk during hip surgery, and how would you assess its function postoperatively?

- The sciatic nerve lies at the posterior aspect of the hip.
- It is derived from L1, L2, S1, S2 and S3 and supplies the short rotators of the hip (obturator internus, the gemelli and quadratus femoris), the hamstrings and half of adductor magnus.
- It also provides motor and sensory function to the leg distal to the knee, except for the area supplied by the saphenous branch of the femoral nerve (which supplies sensation to the medial calf, shin and forefoot).
- Clincal assessment postoperatively is through testing of lateral leg and foot sensation and ankle dorsi- and plantarflexion.

What complications of hip arthroplasty do you know of?

Immediate complications:

- Haemorrhage
- Neurovascular damage
- Fracture.

Early complications:

- Dislocation
- Infection
- Deep venous thrombosis and pulmonary embolism
- Urinary retention.

Late complications:

- Dislocation
- Loosening
- Periprosthetic fracture
- Implant failure/wear
- Inequality in leg length.

26   WRIST LACERATIONS

What elements of the history are important in managing a wrist laceration?

- The epidemiological parameters are particularly important in upper limb trauma – age, hand dominance, occupation and interests may all have an impact on the chosen therapeutic course.
- The mechanism of injury is important: whether this was a fall onto an outstretched hand or deliberate self harm (the flexor tendons often protect the medial nerve at the wrist when lacerations occur in hyperextension or hyperflexion); whether it was cut with a knife or broken glass (with different implications in terms of foreign bodies in the wound and so different infection rates and different wound characteristics).
- Any pre-existing conditions, eg rheumatoid arthritis, carpal tunnel syndrome, triggering of digits.
- Social history (eg smoking) is particularly important, particularly if considering re-implantation surgery.

Can you describe the extensor compartments of the wrist and their contents?

The extensor retinaculum is a thin band of tissue running over the dorsum of the wrist. There are six compartments to this extensor retinaculum – from radial to ulnar they are:

1 Extensor pollicis brevis and abductor pollicis longus
2 Extensor carpi radialis longus and brevis
3 Extensor pollicis longus (via Lister's tubercle)
4 Extensor digitorum communis and extensor indicis
5 Extensor digiti minimi
6 Extensor carpi ulnaris.

How do tendons heal and what technique would you use for a tendon repair?

Tendons heal via a combination of extrinsic and intrinsic cellular activity. The less extrinsic activity, the fewer the adhesions form. It was thought previously that the formation of adhesions was an essential part of tendon healing; recent studies of the intrinsic healing of tendons suggest that this is not the case. The incidence of adhesions is minimised by the use of meticulous surgical technique and early protected mobilisation.

The most commonly used techniques for tendon repair utilise a core suture (eg modified Kessler method) and a running, epi-tendinous peripheral suture to tidy the repair, reduce adhesion formation and add up to 30% of the strength.

27   ACHILLES' TENDON RUPTURE

What is the classic presentation of an Achilles' tendon rupture?

A middle-aged man presents with a sudden sharp pain and 'snap' while undergoing sudden muscular activity: 'It felt like I had been hit in the back of the ankle with the squash racket.' There is pain and inability to stand on tiptoe; there is often a visible deficit in the tendon.

How is it diagnosed and treated?

Diagnosis:

- Thompson/Simmond test is positive when, with the patient prone on the couch with the feet over hanging the edge, compression of the bulk of the calf musculature does not produce plantar flexion.
- Ultrasound scan or magnetic resonance imaging (MRI) will demonstrate the deficit in the Achilles' tendon.

Treatment:

Treatment may be either conservative or surgical (with similar results).

- **Conservative treatment** involves placing the ankle in full plantar flexion, with the knee 45° flexed, in a long-leg plaster of Paris for 4 weeks, then a further 4 weeks in a below-knee plaster of Paris, with slightly less plantar flexion for another 4 weeks. After this, physiotherapy should be instituted and weight-bearing allowed.
- **Surgical treatment** is through placement of an absorbable suture to approximate the tendon ends; the patient should then be managed in a plaster of Paris, much as in the conservative regime, but perhaps with a week less in each plaster. Re-rupture rates are less with surgical treatment.

What is the origin and nerve supply of the gastrocnemius, soleus and plantaris muscles?

- **Gastrocnemius** originates from two heads, the lateral head from the posterior aspect of the lateral condyle of the femur and the medial head from the medial condyle. It inserts via the Achilles' tendon into the posterior aspect of the calcaneum.
- **Soleus** arises from the fibular head and superior quarter of the shaft of the fibula and the soleal line of the tibia and also inserts into the calcaneum via the Achilles' tendon.
- **Plantaris** is a vestigial remnant akin to the palmaris longus in the wrist (with its small belly and long tendon). It arises from the lateral supracondylar aspect

of the femur and the oblique popliteal ligament and inserts into the posteromedial surface of the Achilles' tendon. It is clinically relevant as this muscle is ideal for tendon transfers in the foot and is often torn by athletes with a surprisingly painful presentation.

They are all supplied by the tibial nerve (S1, S2), which is the efferent limb of the ankle reflex.

28   VASECTOMY

What are the important points to remember when obtaining consent from a patient for vasectomy?

- It is an almost irreversible method of sterilisation.
- It is not effective immediately and protection should be used until semen is negative for spermatozoa (it generally takes about 10–20 ejaculations before becoming negative).

How is vasectomy performed?

- Obtain fully informed consent from the patient.
- Prepare the scrotal area and administer local anaesthetic over the site of incision in the scrotum.
- Make a small midline incision over the scrotum.
- Each vas deferens should be exposed and cut, excising a short portion.
- The cut ends are retroflexed and ligated separately.
- Close the wound with absorbable sutures.

What are the specific complications of vasectomy?

- 1% chance of failure
- Spermatocoele
- Psychosexual problems.

29   CIRCUMCISION

What are the indications for circumcision?

- Phimosis
- Paraphimosis
- Recurrent balanitis
- Religious.

How is circumcision performed?

- Obtain fully informed consent and prepare the patient.
- Retract the prepuce.
- Place three haemostats onto the edge of prepuce (one in the midline ventrally and two on either side of midline dorsally).
- Slit the prepuce in the midline dorsally.
- Excise the layers of each flap.
- Trim the inner layer of the prepuce to 3 mm from the corona.
- Approximate the cut edges with absorbable sutures.

What are the specific complications of circumcision?

- Damage to penile shaft or glans
- Bleeding
- Need for repeat circumcision.

30   LAPAROSCOPY

How do you establish a pneumoperitoneum for laparoscopy?

A pneumoperitoneum can be established using either a closed or open method. The **open method** is preferable:

- Obtain fully informed consent.
- Make a small infra-umbilical incision.
- Open the linea alba and peritoneum under direct vision.
- Introduce port into the peritoneal cavity.
- Commence insufflation with carbon dioxide (low pressure and high flow indicate correct positioning of the port in the peritoneal cavity).

What are the reported advantages of laparoscopic surgery over open surgery?

- Less traumatic for patients
- Less postoperative pain
- Improved cosmesis
- Faster postoperative recovery than open surgery
- Reduced adhesion formation
- Shorter stay in hospital and quicker return to work.

(Note that the indications for laparoscopic techniques and their suggested superiority over open techniques have not been fully established for all branches of surgery.)

What ports are used for laparoscopic cholecystectomy?

Four ports are usually used:

- 10-mm umbilical port
- 10-mm subxiphisternal port
- 5-mm anterior axillary line (5 cm below costal margin)
- 5-mm mid-axillary line, parallel to umbilicus.

(Note that 5-mm camera ports are available; and some surgeons perform laparoscopic cholecystectomy using three ports.)

5

PHYSIOLOGY

1   PYREXIA

What conditions can cause a rise in body temperature?

- Infection (swinging pyrexias from abscesses), eg subphrenic abscess
- Inflammation (radiotherapy, chemotherapy, thromboembolism, post-surgical)
- Malignancy
- Drug reactions
- Menstrual cycle
- Malignant hyperpyrexia.

How is pyrexia mediated?

Circulating pyrogens reset the thermostatic mechanism in the hypothalamus:

- **Endogenous pyrogens** (macrophages activate and release interleukin 1 and interleukin 6, promoting the production of endogenous pyrogenic proteins from liver, brain and other organs), or
- **Exogenous pyrogens** (eg bacterial debris).

What is malignant hyperthermia and how is it treated?

- A genetic muscle disorder of muscle, presenting at the time of operation
- Affects 1 in 15,000 paediatric patients and 1 in 40,000 adult patients
- Can have either autosomal dominant or autosomal recessive inheritance (50% have a mutation of the calcium release-channel gene on chromosome 19)
- Acute onset of skeletal muscle rigidity, metabolic acidosis and malignant hyperpyrexia
- Triggered by halogen-containing anaesthetic agents
- Immediate treatment with dantrolene prevents tissue damage and death.

2   CALCIUM

What is the normal plasma concentration of calcium?

The normal range of calcium in plasma is 2.2–2.6 mmol/l (corrected for albumin concentration, as calcium is bound to albumin in blood).

Why is calcium important in the body?

- Calcium is an important second messenger in many cell-signalling pathways.
- It is necessary for blood coagulation, muscle contraction and nerve function.
- Decreased calcium can lead to dysfunction of these systems, eg hypocalcaemia causes excitability of peripheral nerves due to increased neuronal membrane permeability, leading to spontaneous discharge (tetany).

What hormones are responsible for calcium homeostasis and can you briefly describe their actions?

Parathyroid hormone increases serum calcium:

- Stimulates osteclastic activity, leading to bone resorption
- Increases renal phosphate secretion and decreases calcium excretion
- Stimulates 1α-hydroxylase activity in the kidney.

Vitamin D$_3$ (cholecalciferol):

- Derived both from the diet and from ultraviolet light-mediated conversion of 7-dehydrocholesterol in the skin; cholecalciferol is hydroxylated in the liver to 25-hydroxycholecalciferol, which is hydroxylated to 1,25-dihydroxycholecalciferol in the kidney
- 1,25-dihydroxycholecalciferol acts to increase serum calcium and calcification of the bone matrix:
  - stimulates osteoblast proliferation and protein synthesis
  - promotes calcium and phosphate reabsorption in the kidney
  - enhances absorption of calcium and phosphate in the gastrointestinal tract.

Calcitonin decreases serum calcium:

- Inhibits bone resorption through inhibition of osteoclast activity
- Stimulates excretion of calcium, phosphate, sodium and chloride in the kidney.

3   NERVE ACTION POTENTIAL

**Can you draw and label a
nerve action potential?**

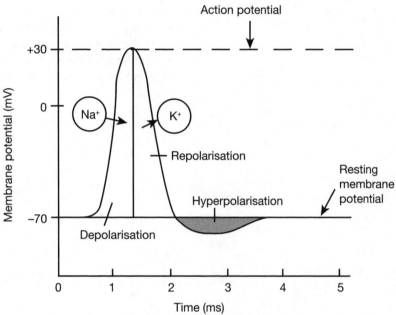

**Can you describe the sequence
of events that occurs during a
nerve action potential?**

- The **resting membrane potential** in a neurone is
  approximately −70 mV (due to the different
  concentrations of sodium, potassium and chloride
  ions inside and outside the cell – sodium is mostly
  intracellular and potassium is mostly extracellular).

- A stimulus activates the fast sodium channels, causing
  rapid influx of sodium ions into the cell and subsequent
  depolarisation of the membrane potential.

- Depolarisation overshoots the zero to +30 mV, which
  inactivates the sodium channels and therefore stops
  further influx of sodium ions.

- Voltage-dependent potassium channels open, causing
  influx of potassium ions and repolarisation back to the
  resting membrane potential of −70 mV.

- When sodium channels are inactivated, the cell is
  refractory to any further stimulus.

- The Na$^+$/K$^+$-ATPase pump plays an important role in
  maintaining intra- and extracellular concentrations of
  sodium and potassium ions.

What influences the speed of neuronal conduction?

- Diameter of the nerve – speed increases with increasing diameter
- Myelination:
  - propagation of the action potential between the nodes of Ranvier (**saltatory conduction**)
  - The **node of Ranvier** is an unmyelinated gap between adjacent Schwann cells.

4   CONTROL OF BLOOD PRESSURE

What mechanisms are involved in the control of blood pressure?

The main mechanisms comprise:

- **Baroreceptors**
- **Autonomic nerve pathways**
- **Vasomotor centre**
- **Cardioinhibitory centre**.

Two additional intrinsic cardiac regulatory mechanisms influence the blood pressure:

- The **Anrep effect** – a response to acute increase in afterload, leads to initial reduction of stroke volume
- The **Bowditch effect** – a response to change in heart rate, the contractility increasing as the rate increases.

What are baroreceptors and where are they found?

Baroreceptors are **stretch receptors** which respond to distension and are present in:

- Carotid sinus
- Aortic arch
- Atrium
- Ventricle.

Other centres intrinsic to baroreceptor function:

- **Vasomotor centre** – a group of neurones in the ventrolateral medulla that maintain the tone of vascular smooth muscle
- **Cardioinhibitory centre** (ventral medulla) – inhibits the vasomotor centre; tone increased by baroreceptor discharge.

What hormonal mechanisms influence the long-term control of blood pressure?

Hormonal mechanisms involved in longer-term blood pressure control:

- Renin–angiotensin system
- Aldosterone
- Vasopressin (ADH)
- Atrial natriuretic peptide (ANP).

5   ARTERIAL WAVEFORM

What are the important features of the arterial waveform?

- Systolic pressure
- Diastolic pressure
- Dicrotic notch
- Pulse pressure
- Mean arterial pressure (the pressure at which the area above the mean equals the area below the mean).

What information can be gained from studying the arterial waveform?

- Arterial blood pressure
- Stroke volume and cardiac output – from the area under the systolic part of the waveform
- Myocardial contractility – from the slope of the upstroke (change in pressure/change in time)
- Outflow resistance – from the slope of diastolic decay:
  - a slow fall suggests vasoconstriction
  - a rapid fall suggests vasodilatation
- Hypovolaemia – suggested by:
  - a low dicrotic notch
  - narrow width of waveform
  - a large variation in peak pressures in patients who are being ventilated.

How does the arterial waveform change in the presence of aortic valve disease?

- Aortic stenosis – slow-rising waveform with a prolonged plateau
- Aortic incompetence – excessive pulse pressure, low diastolic pressure.

6 CARDIAC ACTION POTENTIAL

Can you describe the phases of the cardiac action potential?

- The resting potential of ventricular muscle cells is –90 mV.
- The action potential commences when the membrane of the ventricular muscle is brought to a threshold of around –75 mV by excitation from adjacent muscle cells.
- Once the threshold has been reached, the action potential proceeds in three phases:
  - **phase 1 – rapid depolarisation:** at the threshold, voltage-regulated fast sodium channels open and the membrane rapidly becomes permeable to sodium, resulting in rapid depolarisation of the sarcolemma (duration 3–5 ms)
  - **phase 2 – plateau phase:** as the membrane potential approaches +30 mV, the voltage-regulated sodium channels close. At the same time, slow voltage-regulated calcium channels open. Because calcium channels are slow channels, they remain open for longer (175 ms) and, as a result, the membrane potential remains near 0 mV for an extended period of time known as the 'plateau phase'
  - **phase 3 – repolarisation:** as the plateau continues, the slow calcium channels begin to close and slow potassium channels begin to open. The result is a period of rapid repolarisation that restores the resting potential.
- Following an action potential, the muscle will not respond to a second stimulus – this is called the 'refractory period'. During the **absolute refractory period** the muscle cannot respond at all to any stimulus (duration 200 ms). This is followed by a **relative refractory period**, during which the muscle will only respond to a stimulus that is stronger than normal (duration 50 ms).

What is the main difference between the cardiac action potential and the skeletal muscle action potential?

- Cardiac muscle demonstrates a plateau phase but skeletal muscle does not.
- In a skeletal muscle cell, rapid depolarisation is immediately followed by a period of rapid repolarisation.

Do you know of any drugs that act on the cardiac action potential?

Anti-arrhythmic drugs act by altering the flux of ions across the membranes of excitable cells in the heart. The primary mechanisms of action correspond to the mechanisms used in the **Vaughan Williams' classification system:**

- **Class I drugs** act via inhibition of sodium channels:
  - IA – quinidine and procainamide (prolong repolarisation)
  - IB – lidocaine and phenytoin (shorten repolarisation)
  - IC – flecainide and propafenone (little effect on repolarisation).
- **Class II drugs** block β-adrenergic receptors in the heart:
  - propanolol and esmolol.
- **Class III drugs** inhibit potassium channels:
  - sotalol, amiodarone and bretylium.
- **Class IV drugs** inhibit calcium channels:
  - verapamil and diltiazem.

7   CARDIAC OUTPUT AND OXYGEN FLUX

How do you calculate cardiac output (CO) and what percentage is delivered to each organ system?

CO = stroke volume × rate (usually 70 ml × 70 bpm ≈ 5 l/minute).

Heart	5%
Brain	14%
Muscle	20%
Kidneys	22%
Liver	25%
The rest	14%

How does Starling's law affect contractility and therefore the cardiac output?

- **Starling's law** – the force of myocardial contraction is proportional to initial fibre length.
- If preload is increased, stroke volume will increase, thereby increasing cardiac output (if the rate remains the same).

How do you calculate oxygen flux?

Definition: The oxygen flux, or oxygen delivery (DO_2) is the amount of oxygen delivered to the tissues per unit of time.

$$DO_2 = CO \times \text{arterial } O_2 \text{ content}$$
$$= CO \times (O_2 \text{ bound to Hb} + O_2 \text{ dissolved in plasma})$$
$$= CO \times ((10 \times Hb \times SaO_2 \times 1.34) + (10 \times PaO_2 \times 0.0225))$$

where:

CO	= cardiac output
Hb	= haemoglobin concentration in g/dl
SaO_2	= arterial oxygen saturation of haemoglobin
1.34	= Hüfner's constant
PaO_2	= arterial partial pressure of oxygen
0.0225	= ml of oxygen dissolved/100 ml plasma/kPa (0.003/mmHg).

Normally, the DO_2 is 850–1200 ml/minute.

8   CORONARY CIRCULATION

Can you briefly describe the coronary circulation?

- The **right coronary artery**:
  - arises from the anterior aortic sinus
  - supplies the right ventricle, sinoatrial node and, in 90%, the atrioventricular node and inferior/posterior parts of the left ventricle.
- The **left coronary artery**:
  - arises from the left posterior sinus
  - supplies the anterior wall of the left ventricle and the interventricular septum via the left anterior descending branch
  - supplies the lateral wall of the left ventricle via the circumflex branch.
- The coronary circulation comprises 5% of the cardiac output, ie 250 ml/minute (80 ml/100 g/minute).
- May increase fivefold during exercise.
- Left coronary vessels are compressed by myocardial contraction during systole, so there is only flow to the subendocardium in diastole.
- Atrial and right ventricular flow occur throughout the cardiac cycle.

What factors influence left ventricular perfusion?

Left ventricular blood perfusion is influenced by:

- Difference between aortic end-diastolic pressure and left ventricular end-diastolic pressure
- Duration of diastole (inverse relation to rate)
- Patency of the coronary arteries:
  - autoregulation
  - autonomic neural input
  - coronary spasm/stenosis
  - blood viscosity.

How can coronary blood flow be measured?

- Fick principle (requires coronary sinus catheter)
- Thermodilution technique
- Radioisotope method.

9   BLOOD FLOW IN A VESSEL

What is flow and can you distinguish the different types of flow?

- Flow is the amount of fluid moving per unit of time.
- Flow may be:
  - **laminar**, in which flow is smooth, without eddy currents. Molecules at the periphery move more slowly than those in the centre
  - **turbulent**, when tube is unevenly shaped (eg flow through a narrow orifice); or during laminar flow when flow velocity exceeds critical velocity.
- **Reynold's number** describes the relationship between tube and fluid characteristics and the velocity at which turbulent flow occurs:
  - Reynold's number <2000 – flow likely to be laminar
  - Reynold's number >3000 – flow likely to be turbulent

How do you measure flow?

- Gaseous flow – flow meters
- Liquid flow:
  - dilution techniques
  - electromagnetic flow measurement
  - Fick principle.

How is flow related to the radius of a tube?

Flow is proportional to R^4 (radius to the power of 4).

The **Hagen–Poiseuille equation describes laminar flow:**

$$Flow = (P \times R^4 \times \pi)/(8 \times \eta \times L)$$

where:

P = pressure gradient across the tube
R = radius of the tube
η = viscosity of the tube
L = length of the tube.

10   CARBON DIOXIDE

How is carbon dioxide transported in the blood?

Carbon dioxide is transported:

- As bicarbonate (60%)
- Coupled to amino group of haemoglobin (30%)
- Dissolved in plasma (10%).

What are the effects of hypercarbia?

Definition: $Pa_{CO_2} > 6$ kPa.

Central nervous system effects:

- Increases cerebral blood flow (increased hydrogen ions)
- Stimulates sympathetic nervous system
- Carbon dioxide narcosis at levels ≥12 kPa.

Respiratory system effects:

- Carbon dioxide stimulates respiration at levels ≤13 kPa, above this level, it acts as a depressant
- Increases peripheral vascular resistance.

Cardiovascular system effects:

- Myocardial depressant (effect blunted due to sympathetic stimulation initially, but at higher levels cardiac output is severely affected)
- Arrhythmias.

Renal effects:

- Constriction of glomerular afferent arterioles, leading to reduced urine output with high levels of carbon dioxide.

What are the clinical features of carbon dioxide retention?

- Flushed skin
- Characteristic coarse flap of the hands (asterixis)
- Bounding pulse
- Muscle twitching
- Hypertension
- Ventricular ectopics
- Convulsions
- Coma.

11 LUNG FUNCTION TESTS

What is the peak expiratory flow rate (PEFR)?

Definition: Maximal rate of air flow during a sudden forced expiration (litres/minute).

- Normal female PEFR: 350–500 litres/minute
- Normal male PEFR: 450–700 litres/minute
- Reduced in obstructive disease, eg asthma.

Can you define the values obtained in spirometry?

FEV: forced expiratory volume; volume of gas forcibly exhaled from full inspiration.

FEV_1: forced expiratory volume exhaled in 1 second (reduced in obstructive pulmonary disease).

FVC: forced vital capacity; largest volume if air forcibly expired after maximum inspiration (reduced in restrictive disease, if supine, elderly, muscle weakness, emphysema).

FEV_1/**FVC:** expressed as a percentage; normal is >70% (reduced in obstructive disease; increased/normal in restrictive disease).

What is lung compliance?

Definition: Volume change per unit of pressure change, ie a measure of distensibility.

- Normal lung compliance is 150–200 ml/cmH$_2$O.
- Can be divided into:
  - **static compliance**, ie alveolar distensibility (reduced in pulmonary fibrosis and pulmonary oedema)
  - **dynamic compliance** – related to airway resistance (decreased in chronic bronchitis).

12 OXYGEN DISSOCIATION CURVE

What is the relationship between the Po$_2$ of blood and the oxygen saturation of haemoglobin?

This is explained by the **oxygen dissociation curve**:

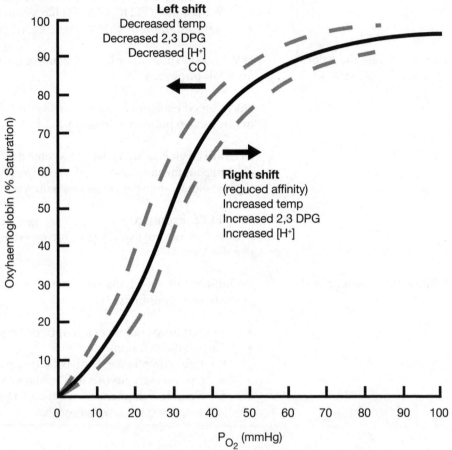

There are three reference points on the curve:

- P50 = 3.6 kPa
- P75 = 5.3 kPa
- P100 = 13.3 kPa

How do clinical conditions affect the shape of the curve?

The **curve is shifted to the right** (ie decreased affinity for oxygen) by:

- Acidosis
- Increased 2,3-DPG
- Increased temperature
- Hypercapnia (Bohr effect).

The **curve is shifted to the left** (ie increased oxygen affinity) by:

- Fetal haemoglobin (HbF)
- Decreased 2,3-DPG
- Alkalosis
- Methaemoglobinaemia
- Carbon monoxide poisoning
- Hypothermia
- Hypocapnia.

What is the importance of the sigmoid shaped curve?

- A fall in Po_2 is tolerated provided the saturation remains above 90% (ie the flat part of the curve).
- Increasing the Po_2 above normal has little effect unless hyperbaric oxygen is used, when the amount of oxygen in solution in the plasma becomes significant.
- On the steep part of the curve, small decreases in Po_2 lead to large falls in saturation (ie oxygen content).

13   MUSCLE

What are the different types of muscle found in the body?

- **Skeletal** (striated):
  - long, cylindrical, non-branching fibres
  - parallel or oblique
- **Smooth** (non-striated):
  - narrow, parallel, spindle-shaped cells
  - slow but sustained contraction
  - autonomic nerves; gap junctions
- **Cardiac** (striated):
  - less powerful than skeletal muscle but more prone to fatigue.

What is the structure of skeletal muscle and how does it contract?

- Epimysium (around muscle bundles)
- Perimysium (around muscle fascicles)
- Endomysium (around individual myofibrils)
- Sarcomeres contain actin (I) and mysosin (H); actin is attached to Z lines and myosin is attached to M lines.

Acetylcholine is released at the synapse when the depolarisation impulse arrives at the neuromuscular junction. This leads to a cascade of events which results in depolarisation of the sarcoplasmic reticulum and release of calcium. The calcium binds to troponin on the thin filaments, changing the position of tropomyosin on the thin filaments. This exposes actin and leads to the formation of cross-bridges.

What is the difference between the muscles of marathon runners and the muscles of sprinters?

Marathon runners have predominantly **slow-twitch fibres** (red):

- Aerobic – more mitochondria, enzymes and triglycerides
- Low concentration of glycolytic enzymes (ATPase) and glycogen
- Best remembered by the expression 'slow red ox'.

Sprinters have predominantly **fast-twitch fibres** (white):

- Larger, stronger motor units
- ATP–creatine phosphate system.

14   PERIPHERAL NERVES

What are the different layers within a peripheral nerve?

External epineurium surrounding **internal epineurium**, surrounding **fascicular groups** (consisting of **perineurium**), surrounding **fascicles** (consisting of **endoneurium**), surrounding **nerve fibres** (consisting of **Schwann cell/myelin sheath**), surrounding the **axon**.

What physiological changes occur in the nerve following injury?

- Proximal stump undergoes Wallerian degeneration to the proximal node of Ranvier.
- Cell body increases RNA synthesis.
- Multiple axonal sprouts – 'growth cones' with filipodia.
- Distal stump undergoes Wallerian degeneration (leaving empty neural tubes, Schwann cells and basal lamina).
- Axonal sprouts reaching distal Schwann cells continue to grow (1 mm/day), others degenerate.

How do you classify nerve injuries?

- **Neurapraxia:**
  - reversible conduction block
  - local ischaemia and selective demyelination of axon sheath
  - good prognosis
- **Axonotmesis:**
  - disruption of axon and myelin sheath, leaving epineurium intact
  - fair prognosis
- **Neuronotmesis:**
  - complete nerve division with disruption of the endoneurium
  - poor prognosis.

15   CARTILAGE

Can you name the different types of cartilage?

- Physeal cartilage – growth plate
- Fibrocartilage – tendon and ligament insertions into bone, healing articular cartilage
- Elastic – trachea
- Fibroelastic – menisci
- Hyaline – articular cartilage.

What is the composition of articular cartilage?

- **Water** (65%–80%):
  - allows nutrition and lubrication
  - shifts in and out in response to stress
- **Collagen** (10%–20%):
  - 90%–95% is type II collagen
  - provides framework and tensile strength
- **Proteoglycans** (10%–15%):
  - protein polysaccharides produced by chondrocytes
  - provides compressive strength of cartilage
- **Chondrocytes** (5%):
  - protein synthesis – collagen, proteoglycans and enzymes.

If cartilage is avascular, aneural and alymphatic, how does it heal after injury?

Superficial injury:

- Does not cross the tidemark
- Chondrocytes proliferate but cartilage does not heal.

Deep injury:

- Extends below the tidemark
- May heal with fibrocartilage
- Fibrocartilage is formed by differentiation of marrow mesenchymal stem cells into cells capable of producing fibrocartilage.

16   BONE

What are the different types of bone?

- **Cortical bone:**
  - tightly packed osteons structured along lines of stress
  - slow turnover
- **Cancellous bone:**
  - less dense and undergoes more remodelling
  - high turnover rate
- **Lamellar** versus **woven** bone.

Can you describe the microscopic composition of bone?

Cells:

- Osteoblasts
- Osteoclasts
- Osteocytes
- Lining cells
- Osteoprogenitor cells.

Matrix:

- Organic (40%):
  - collagen (type I)
  - proteoglycans
  - matrix proteins, eg osteocalcin
  - growth factors and cytokines
- Inorganic (60%):
  - calcium hydroxyapatite
  - osteocalcium phosphate (brushite).

What are the different stages of fracture healing?

- **Haematoma formation**
- **Inflammation**
- **Repair:**
  - soft callus (from proliferating osteogenic cells on periosteal and endosteal surfaces)
  - hard callus (callus stiffens progressively as the woven bone mineralises into lamellar bone)
- **Remodelling** (stress stimulates thicker lamellae to form; medullary cavity reforms from callus).

17   TEMPERATURE REGULATION

How are changes in body temperature detected?

- The hypothalamus and spinal cord have thermoreceptors for core temperature.
- Skin has receptors for peripheral temperature.
- All signals are sent to the hypothalamus.

Can you describe the body's response to hypothermia?

The response is mediated via the autonomic and somatic nervous systems:

- **Somatic response:**
  - increased voluntary muscle activity and curling up
  - shivering (can increase basal metabolic rate (BMR) fourfold)
- **Autonomic response:**
  - vasoconstriction (directly, via skin thermoreceptors)
  - hair stands up (horripilation)
  - sweat glands inhibited
  - brown fat activated (in infants).

How do you manage a hypothermic patient?

- Check airway, give oxygen and ventilate if needed.
- Set up an intravenous infusion of warm fluids and send off bloods.
- Monitor the patient:
  - accurate per rectal temperature probe
  - ECG – J waves and arrhythmias
  - urinary catheter.
- Actively rewarm at half a degree Celsius per hour unless rapidly cooled.
- Thermal blanket, Bair Hugger®, infusion of warm fluids into the peritoneal cavity or bladder, haemodialysis, cardiopulmonary bypass.
- Investigate the reason for the hypothermia and deal with this (including home or social situation if applicable).

18   HYPONATRAEMIA

What are the symptoms of hyponatraemia?

Definition: Plasma sodium <135 mmol/l.

Symptoms: headache, nausea, confusion, coma, convulsions (symptoms depend on the rate as well as the magnitude of the fall in plasma sodium).

What are the causes of hyponatraemia?

- Water excess – increased intake, reduced excretion, cardiac/hepatic/renal failure, nephrotic syndrome
- Water deficiency with greater relative sodium deficiency – diuretic therapy, hypoadrenalism, nephritis, renal tubular acidosis
- Other causes – diarrhoea, vomiting, pancreatitis.

How would you treat hyponatraemia?

- Correction should be gradual (otherwise, problems that may arise include subdural haemorrhage, pontine lesions, cardiac failure); correct at a rate of 5–10 mmol/day (faster if plasma sodium <120 mmol/l)
- Treat underlying cause
- Water restriction
- Intravenous normal saline
- Diuretics (eg furosemide)
- Intravenous hypertonic saline (controversial).

19   HEPATIC FUNCTION AND HEPATIC FAILURE

What are the functions of the liver?

- Production of bile
- Excretion of bilirubin
- Storage of glycogen
- Production of plasma proteins
- Production of clotting factors
- Metabolism of drugs
- Formation of urea from ammonia
- Formation of acetoacetic acid
- Kupffer cells (macrophage function)
- Blood reservoir and production of heat.

What complications of liver disease are relevant in the perioperative period?

- Bleeding:
  - prolonged prothrombin time (PT)
  - thrombocytopenia
  - oesophageal and gastric varices
- Encephalopathy
- Hypoglycaemia
- Ascites due to portal hypertension, sodium and water retention and low albumin
- Depressed immune function
- Renal failure.

What is Child's classification?

Child's classification is a system of classifying the risk of mortality for surgery and anaesthesia in hepatic failure, based on:

- Bilirubin
- Albumin
- Prothrombin time
- Ascites
- Encephalopathy
- Nutrition.

20   RENAL FUNCTION

What are the functions of the kidney?

- Filtration of plasma, excretion of waste products of metabolism, and maintenance of water and electrolyte homeostasis
- Secretion of renin and erythropoietin
- Metabolism and excretion of drugs
- Formation of 1,25-dihydroxycholecalciferol (calcium homeostasis).

What is the glomerular filtration rate (GFR)?

Definition: Volume (in ml) of plasma filtered by the kidneys per minute (normal is 120 ml/minute).

How do you measure GFR?

The GFR is measured by infusion of a substance that is freely filtered and neither reabsorbed nor secreted by renal tubules:

The basic formula for clearance (Cx) of a substance x is:

GFR (Cx) = (urine concentration of x (mg/dl) × urine volume/time)/plasma concentration of x

Inulin can be used but is difficult to measure.

An alternative is to use creatinine clearance (approximates to the GFR), averaged over 24 hours (normal range is 90–130 ml/minute).

21 RENIN–ANGIOTENSIN–ALDOSTERONE SYSTEM

What is renin and what stimulates its release?

- Renin is a proteolytic enzyme (molecular weight 40,000 Da)
- Synthesised and stored in the juxtaglomerular apparatus
- Released in response to decreases in circulating volume:
  - decreased afferent arteriolar pressure
  - decreased sodium delivery at the macula densa.

What are the actions of angiotensin II?

- Vasoconstriction – intrarenal and systemic
- Increased proximal tubular sodium reabsorption
- Aldosterone release from the adrenal cortex
- Increased distal tubular sodium reabsorption
- Stimulates thirst
- Antidiuretic hormone release – leads to water retention.

What are the causes of hyperaldosteronism?

Primary – adrenal cortical tumour (Conn's syndrome).

Secondary:

- Pregnancy
- Heart failure
- Chronic diuretic therapy
- Dietary salt restriction
- Cirrhosis with ascites
- Nephrosis.

22   STARLING'S FORCES

How do Starling's forces affect the capillary level?

Definition: Factors determining the movement of fluid across the capillary wall endothelium.

Movement of water into the interstitium is produced by the hydrostatic pressure gradient and counteracted by the colloid osmotic gradient.

How do these forces interact?

P_c = capillary hydrostatic pressure (varies from artery to vein)
P_{if} = interstitial hydrostatic pressure
π_p = oncotic pressure due to plasma proteins (28 mmHg)
π_{if} = oncotic pressure due to interstitial proteins (3 mmHg)
Net filtration = $(P_c - P_{if}) - (\pi_p - \pi_{if})$

What factors can lead to the development of oedema?

Definition: Generalised or local excess of extracellular fluid.

- Hypoproteinaemia and decreased plasma oncotic pressure
- Increased hydrostatic pressure (cardiac failure)
- Venous or lymphatic obstruction
- Salt/water retention (renal impairment/failure)
- Leaky capillary endothelium (inflammation, allergic reactions)
- Direct instillation.

23   THYROID HORMONES

What hormones are produced by the thyroid gland and how are they produced?

Hormones:

- Tri-iodothyronine (T3)
- Thyroxine (T4).

Production:

- Active transport of iodide across the basement membrane into the thyroid follicular cell (iodide trapping)
- Oxidation of iodide and iodination of tyrosyl residues in thyroglobulin, coupling of iodotyrosine molecules within thyroglobulin to form T3 and T4
- T3 and T4 released from the thyroid by proteolysis reach the bloodstream where they are bound to thyroid hormone-binding proteins
- Thyroxine-binding globulin (TBG) normally accounts for 75% of the bound hormone.

How is the production of these hormones regulated?

- All the reactions necessary for the production of T3 and T4 are influenced by thyroid-stimulating hormone (TSH).
- Pituitary TSH secretion is controlled by a negative-feedback mechanism modulated by the circulating levels of free T4 and free T3 – increased levels of free T4 and free T3 inhibit the release of TSH; and decreased levels of free T4 and free T3 stimulate the release of TSH.
- Thyrotrophin-releasing hormone (TRH), synthesised by the hypothalamus, also influences the secretion of TSH.
- When TRH is released into the portal system between the hypothalamus and pituitary, it stimulates the release of TSH from anterior pituitary thyrotropic cells.
- An adequate supply of iodine is essential for normal thyroid hormone production.

What are the effects of thyroid hormones on the body?

- **Metabolism** – T3 increases oxygen consumption and heat production, which contribute to increased basal metabolic rate.
- **Brain** – fetal brain development and skeletal maturation.
- **Cardiovascular** – T3 improves cardiac muscle contractility.
- **Autonomic nervous system:**
  - increase the number of β-adrenergic receptors in heart muscle, skeletal muscle, adipose tissue and lymphocytes

- • stimulate hepatic gluconeogenesis and glycogenolysis as well as intestinal absorption of glucose.
- • **Gastrointestinal/hepatic** – stimulate gut motility.
- • **Bone** – increase bone turnover.

24   ACID–BASE BALANCE

What is an acid, a base and a buffer?

- An acid is a proton donor.
- A base is a proton acceptor.
- A buffer is a combination of a weak acid and its conjugate base. It works best at a pH equal to its pKa, ie when it is maximally dissociated.

What is acidosis and how is it classified?

- Acidosis occurs when the pH of the arterial blood is less than 7.35.
- It may be classified into metabolic and non-metabolic causes.
- This distinction is made via the **anion gap** which is defined as the sum of the major cations (ie sodium and potassium) minus the sum of the major anions (bicarbonate and chloride). The normal range for the anion gap is between 12 mmol/l and 20 mmol/l.
- An **acidosis with a normal anion gap** results from the replacement of bicarbonate by chloride, caused by:
  - gastrointestinal losses – diarrhoea, pancreatic fistula, ileostomy
  - renal – renal tubular acidosis types III and IV.
- An **acidosis with an increased anion gap** signifies that there has been addition of exogenous or endogenous fixed acids, as in:
  - lactic acidosis
  - diabetic ketoacidosis.

What are the major buffering systems in the human body?

The major buffer in the blood is the bicarbonate system. Others include the phosphate and the ammonia systems. The proteins in the body also buffer changes in pH (eg globin chains in the blood and cytoplasmic proteins intracellularly). These factors make up the immediate buffers.

Acutely, the respiratory system can assist in pH homeostasis by reducing the concentration of volatile acid (by blowing off carbon dioxide).

In chronic states, buffering occurs in the kidney, where filtered bicarbonate and phosphate are replaced with regenerated bicarbonate, and new bicarbonate is formed from glutamine. Bone also buffers protons in exchange with anions from its mineral matrix, and the liver can secrete new bicarbonate and ammonia, again from glutamine.

25   SERUM LIPIDS

What is atheroma?

Atheroma is a localised intimal collection of foamy macro-phages, fibroblasts and lipid deposits, associated with smooth-muscle hyperplasia, within large and medium-sized arteries.

The major **risk factors** for atheroma formation are hyper-lipidaemia, hypertension, diabetes and smoking; other risk factors are male gender, a family history and genetic hyper-lipidaemia.

There are three **theories on atheroma formation**:

1   **Encrustation** – the lipid is derived from intimal thrombus.
2   **Proliferation** – PDGF and low-density lipoprotein stimulate smooth muscle hyperplasia.
3   **Imbibition** – hypertension forces circulating lipoproteins across the vessel wall.

What are the complications of atheroma?

- Gradual obstruction of the vessel lumen, leading to ischaemia
- Sudden occlusion of the vessel lumen by rupture of a plaque or haemorrhage into a plaque
- Downstream occlusion by embolism of lipid from the plaque, or by embolism of thrombus from the surface of the plaque
- Rupture or aneurysm formation within the vessel.

What are lipoproteins and how are they classified?

Definition: Lipoproteins are spherical particles made up of apoproteins, phospholiplids, triglycerides, cholesterol and cholesterol esters. The concentration of cholesterol varies in different lipoproteins.

Lipoproteins are classified by their density (via separation in an ultracentrifuge):

- **High-density lipoproteins** (HDL):
  - contain less than 25% cholesterol
  - the 'good' lipoprotein in terms of reducing atheroma
  - represent the major pool of apoproteins and transport cholesterol from the periphery to the liver for excretion and metabolism
- **Low-density lipoproteins** (LDL):
  - contain approximately 70% cholesterol
  - the 'bad' lipoprotein (they are the main transport medium for cholesterol from the liver)

- - taken up by many cells that express the LDL receptor; cleared from the blood by the liver for recycling
  - **Very low-density lipoproteins** (VLDL):
    - contain only 25% cholesterol but are 60% triglyceride
    - secreted by the liver to carry lipids to the periphery
    - release triglycerides to become the short-lived 'intermediate-density lipoproteins' (IDL), which then become LDL
  - **Chylomicrons:**
    - largest particles, containing only 10% cholesterol but almost 90% triglycerides
    - formed in the gut and transport lipids to the body
    - triglycerides are removed from them (to feed muscle and to be stored in adipose tissue) to form chylomicron remnants that are high in cholesterol and taken up by the liver.

26   SECONDARY MESSENGERS

What is a secondary messenger?

The primary messenger is a hormone and its secondary messenger is a chemical produced within the cell by the action of the hormone on the cell membrane.

What secondary messengers do you know?

- Cyclic adenosine monophosphate (cAMP)
- Diacylglycerol (DAG)
- Inositol triphosphate (IP3).

Can you describe the secondary messengers at receptor level in the autonomic nervous system?

The autonomic nervous system is divided into two systems:

1. The **sympathetic system** has α and β receptors and each of these has a number of subsets:
   - α_1-receptor stimulation causes an increase in IP3 and DAG (via phospholipase C activation).
   - α_2-receptor stimulation leads to a decrease in cAMP (via inhibition of phospholipase C).
   - β_1 and β_2 receptors both increase cAMP (via stimulation of adenyl cylase).
2. The **parasympathetic system** utilises muscarinic and nicotinic receptors:
   - Muscarinic receptors use a G-protein coupled mechanism but the secondary messenger is unknown.
   - Nicotinic receptors do not have a secondary messenger as they are directly linked to ion channels (eg the neuromuscular end plate).
   - Nicotinic receptors are also found at the postganglionic membrane of both the sympathetic and parasympathetic nervous systems.

27   NEUROMUSCULAR JUNCTION

What do you understand about the neuromuscular junction?

- The neuromuscular junction is the synapse between the presynaptic motor neurone and the postsynaptic muscle membrane.
- The axon divides into terminal buttons that invaginate into the muscle fibre.
- The **synaptic cleft** is 50–70 nm wide and filled with extracellular fluid.
- The orifices (synaptic clefts) lie opposite the release points for acetylcholine and contain high concentrations of acetylcholinesterase.
- The action potential conducted along the motor nerve causes depolarisation and an influx of calcium.
- The influx of calcium stimulates the release of acetylcholine from storage vesicles into the synapse; acetylcholine binds to nicotinic receptors on the motor end plate.
- Stimulation of the acetylcholine receptor results in opening of sodium channels (and some potassium channels), and influx of sodium and potassium into the cell results in depolarisation.
- Depolarisation is called the **end plate potential** – if the end plate potential is sufficiently large, an **action potential** is produced and muscle contraction occurs.
- Acetylcholine is hydrolysed by acetylcholinesterase and the product choline is taken back up through the presynaptic membrane to re-produce acetylcholine.

Do you know any toxins that block neuromuscular transmission?

Botulinum toxin:

- Botulinum toxin is an exotoxin produced by *Clostridium botulinum*, a Gram-positive spore-forming bacillus.
- The toxin is internalised in the presynaptic membrane and binds to the vesicle membrane.
- This prevents the release of the vesicle and therefore acetylcholine at the neuromuscular junction.

Do you know any anaesthetic agents that block neuromuscular transmission?

Depolarising muscle relaxants:

- Produce what appears to be a persistent depolarisation of the neuromuscular junction.
- Cause depolarisation by mimicking the effect of acetylcholine but without being rapidly hydrolysed by acetylcholinesterase.
- Examples include suxamethonium and decamethonium.

Non-depolarising muscle relaxants:

- Compete with acetylcholine for nicotinic receptor-binding sites.
- The blockade is competitive, so muscle paralysis occurs gradually.
- Examples include tubocurarine, atracurium and vecuronium.

28   BILE SALTS AND GALLSTONES

What are the functions of bile salts?

- Act as a detergent, emulsifying fats to facilitate their absorption.
- Contain bicarbonate, which neutralises the acidic contents of gastric juice.
- Provide a route for the excretion of bile pigments, steroids and drugs.
- Facilitate the absorption of fat-soluble vitamins (A, D, E and K).

What different types of gallstones do you know and what are they made from?

There three common varieties of stones:

1   **Mixed** (75%):
    - most common type, often multiple, pale and faceted
    - major component is cholesterol
    - cut surface is laminated with alternate dark and light zones of pigment and cholesterol respectively.
2   **Cholesterol** (20%):
    - often large solitary stones
    - cut surface shows crystals radiating from the centre of the stone
    - surface is yellow and greasy to touch.
3   **Pigment** (5%):
    - small, black, irregular and multiple; associated with haemolytic anaemia
    - composed of calcium bilirubinate and calcium carbonate.

What is a 'strawberry gallbladder'?

When cholesterol precipitates from bile on the gallbladder wall, it forms yellow submucous collections of cholesterol with an appearance similar to a strawberry skin. These are usually associated with cholesterol stones.

29   GASTRIC FUNCTION

What are the functions of the stomach?

- Produces hydrochloric acid, pepsin, intrinsic factor and mucus secretions.
- Acts as a reservoir to allow the process of digestion to occur.
- The mixing of food and gastric juices produces **chyme**, which travels to the small intestine for further digestion and absorption.
- Release of the hormone **gastrin** (from the G cells of pyloric glands).

How is gastric acid secretion regulated?

There are three phases in gastric acid production:

1   **Cephalic phase:** Acid is initially produced by the sight, smell, taste and thought of food. It is vagally mediated and the acetylcholine released directly stimulates the parietal cells to produce acid. It also stimulates acid secretion indirectly by releasing gastrin from the G cells of the gastric mucosa.

2   **Gastric phase:** The contact of food with the stomach produces gastrin by mechanical and chemical stimulation. The distension of the body or antrum of the stomach is the mechanical stimulus and the products of digestion (eg amino acids) in the antrum cause gastrin release and hence acid production. The presence of food also excites vagal reflexes to stimulate parietal cells to produce acid. When the buffering capacity of the stomach is saturated and the pH falls, there is inhibition of further acid release.

3   **Intestinal phase:** This phase is mainly associated with the inhibition of gastric acid production and neutralisation of acid when entering the duodenum. This is brought about by the presence of acid, fat digestion products and hypertonicity in the duodenum and proximal jejunum. Acid in the duodenum causes the release of **secretin**, which inhibits gastrin release. Fatty acids cause the release of **cholecystokinin** and **gastric inhibitory peptide,** inhibiting gastric acid secretion by parietal cells.

Which tumour can lead to the development of multiple severe peptic ulcers?

Gastrinoma:

- Due to gastrin-secreting adenomas in the pancreas, duodenum, stomach or elsewhere (eg cystadenoma of the ovary) or simple islet-cell hyperplasia.
- 50%–60% of tumours are malignant and 50% are multiple.

- 30% of cases are associated with the autosomal dominant disorder of **multiple endocrine neoplasia** (MEN 1).
- Overproduction of gastrin leads to **Zollinger–Ellison syndrome**, with widespread peptic ulceration and diarrhoea.

30   MECHANICS OF RESPIRATION

What do you understand by the term 'mechanical breathing'?

Definition: The movements of the thorax that enable ventilation of the lung tissue. There are two types of mechanical breathing:

- **Quiet breathing**, which occurs at rest
- **Forced breathing**, which occurs during exercise or when there is diseased lung tissue, requiring extra ventilation to oxygenate the blood.

Can you describe the mechanical process of breathing?

There are two phases of breathing:

Inspiration:

- The thorax expands in three dimensions.
- During inspiration, the thorax expands mainly in its vertical diameter, as a result of the contraction and flattening of the diaphragm (known as **diaphragmatic breathing**) supplied by the phrenic nerve (C3, C4, C5).
- **Thoracic breathing** involves movement of the upper two to seven ribs in a 'pump-handle' action, which increases the anteroposterior diameter of the chest.
- The lower eight to twelve ribs move in a 'bucket-handle' manner, thereby increasing the lateral diameter of the chest.
- These movements of the ribs are brought about by the contraction of the external and internal oblique intercostal muscles.
- This causes the pressure in the pleural cavity to drop to -4 mmHg, causing air to flow into the lungs down the pressure gradient.
- The **accessory muscles of respiration** are used in forced and in deep inspiration (sternocleidomastoid, scalene muscles, pectoralis minor and major and serratus anterior).

Expiration:

- Elastic recoil of the lungs and chest wall rather than muscular contraction is responsible for quiet expiration.
- Forced expiration involves the abdominal muscles and latissimus dorsi.

What is lung compliance and in what situations is it decreased?

- Compliance refers to the elasticity of the lungs.
- Defined as change in lung volume per unit change in pressure.
- Poor lung compliance occurs in:
  - lung disease, eg in pulmonary fibrosis
  - disease of the chest wall, eg in thoracic scoliosis.

6
CRITICAL CARE

1   ACUTE LUNG INJURY

What is 'acute lung injury' (ALI)?

Acute respiratory failure characterised by:

- Diffuse pulmonary infiltrates
- Progressive hypoxaemia
- Reduced lung compliance
- Normal hydrostatic pressures.

Diagnostic criteria:

- Bilateral pulmonary infiltrates on chest X-ray
- Pulmonary capillary wedge pressure <18 mmHg
- PaO_2/FiO_2 <300 mmHg (40 kPa) = ALI
- PaO_2/FiO_2 <200 mmHg (26 kPa) = ARDS.

The most severe form of ALI is acute respiratory distress syndrome (ARDS).

What is the pathology seen in ALI/ARDS?

- Caused by a stimulus to the local or systemic inflammatory response.
- **Causes** include:
  - shock
  - sepsis, particularly Gram-negative bacteria
  - haemorrhage
  - trauma – multisystem trauma, direct lung trauma, near drowning, smoke inhalation
  - cerebral – head injury, cerebral haemorrhage
  - embolism – fat, air, amniotic fluid
  - others – acute pancreatitis, disseminated intravascular coagulation, cardiopulmonary bypass, massive blood transfusion, eclampsia, oxygen toxicity.
- Occurs 12–72 hours after precipitating insult.
- Early changes – interstitial and alveolar oedema, containing red blood cells, white blood cells, proteins and hyaline membrane.
- Late changes – interstitial fibrosis with proliferation of alveolar type II cells, obstruction and destruction of the microcirculation of the lung.
- Multiple-organ failure is a common outcome.

What are the principles of treating ALI/ARDS?

- Treatment is primarily supportive.
- Treat the underlying cause if possible.
- Try to maintain PaO_2 >60 mmHg, but try to keep FiO_2 between 0.5 and 0.6 (to avoid oxygen toxicity).
- Ventilation strategies:
  - positive end-expiratory pressure (PEEP)

- inverse ventilation ratio (inspiratory phase > expiratory phase) – re-opens collapsed alveloli
- prone-position ventilation.
- Drugs:
  - none conclusively shown to be of benefit
  - nitric oxide – reduces pulmonary hypertension, reduces shunting, improves gas exchange
  - prostacyclin
  - surfactant
  - corticosteroids.

2   FLUID AND ELECTROLYTE BALANCE

What are the clinical signs of dehydration?

- Dry mucous membranes
- Decreased skin turgor
- Tachycardia
- Hypotension
- Reduced urine output
- Reduced level of consciousness
- Sunken fontanelles in young children.

Following a laparotomy, what losses need to be taken into account and how do you calculate these?

Basic fluid requirements	25 ml/kg/day
Insensible losses	20 ml/hour
Pyrexia	add 10 ml/hour for each degree above 37 °C
Anticipated ileus	add 20 ml/hour first day
Third space losses	add 40 ml/hour first day
Consider other losses, eg bleeding	

What does Hartmann's solution contain?

Na^+	131 mmol/l
Cl^-	111 mmol/l
K^+	5 mmol/l
Ca^{2+}	2 mmol/l
HCO_3^-	29 mmol/l (as lactate)
Osmolality	278 mosmol/l

Maintains composition of extracellular environment when large volumes of intravenous fluids are required over a short period of time (used in ATLS protocol).

3   ARTERIAL BLOOD GASES

How do you take an arterial blood sample?

- Clean procedure
- Radial artery (preferably the non-dominant hand – use Allen's test to ensure dual blood supply to the hand) or femoral artery
- 2 ml heparinised syringe
- Gentle aspiration after seeing flashback
- Keep sample cool until analysis
- Firm pressure on artery to prevent haematoma.

Can you interpret the two blood gas sample results?

Sample 1
pH 7.081
P_{CO_2} 2.76 kPa
P_{O_2} 14.10 kPa
Base excess −22.4 mmol/l
HCO_3^- 8.4 mmol/l
Sa_{O_2} 94.9%
Haemoglobin 13.2 g/dl

Sample 2
pH 7.275
P_{CO_2} 12.98 kPa
P_{O_2} 4.44 kPa
Base excess 15.8 mmol/l
HCO_3^- 33.9 mmol/l
Sa_{O_2} 55.1%
Haemoglobin 18.2 g/dl

Sample 1

Metabolic acidosis, low P_{CO_2}, indicating compensatory respiratory alkalosis to moderate the metabolic acidosis, eg diabetic ketoacidosis.

Sample 2

Respiratory acidosis, high bicarbonate and base excess, suggesting metabolic compensation. The high haemoglobin and hypoxia suggest chronic respiratory failure.

What are the potential errors in arterial blood gas sampling?

- Over-heparinisation of the sample (increased acidosis)
- Air in the syringe (raises P_{O_2}, lowers P_{CO_2})
- Delayed analysis without cooling (decreased P_{O_2} and pH, increased P_{CO_2}, due to metabolism by white cells).

4   HYPOXIA

How do you classify hypoxia?

Hypoxaemic hypoxia – reduced PaO_2 due to hypoventilation, diffusion impairment, shunt, $\dot{V}/\dot{Q}$ mismatch.

Stagnant hypoxia – inadequate blood supply to an organ; PaO_2 and haemoglobin may be normal.

Cytotoxic hypoxia – normal oxygen delivery but cells prevented from utilising it (cytochrome poisoning).

Anaemic hypoxia – PaO_2 normal, haemoglobin low.

Can you suggest methods of supplementary oxygen delivery?

Nasal cannula	30%–40%
Face mask	up to 50%
Venturi mask (fixed performance)	up to 60%
Reservoir bag	up to 100%

What are the problems and risks associated with oxygen therapy?

- Reduced hypoxic ventilatory drive (be aware of this in COPD)
- Pulmonary toxicity (increased free oxygen radicals; decreased surfactant and compliance)
- Atelectasis
- Fire risk.

(See also Question 6, Oxygen delivery.)

5   SHOCK

What is the initial treatment of hypovolaemic shock?

- **Airway** – oxygen via face mask
- **Breathing**
- **Circulation** (with haemorrhage control) – two large-bore cannulae for intravenous access (antecubital fossa)
- Crystalloid/colloid, blood, clotting products (if large transfusion required)
- Patient positioning (head down)
- Crossmatch as necessary
- Investigations (FBC, U&Es, clotting screen).

How do you assess adequate resuscitation?

Assess:

- Blood pressure
- Heart rate
- Capillary refill (peripheral perfusion)
- Temperature (peripheral perfusion)
- Urine output
- Blood gases:
  - lactate
  - base excess.

If available, consider:

- Central venous pressure monitoring
- Pulmonary capillary wedge pressure (PCWP).

What are the different types of shock?

- **Hypovolaemic shock**, eg secondary to trauma
- **Cardiogenic shock**, eg secondary to myocardial infarction
- **Distributive shock** – sepsis, neurogenic, anaphylaxis
- **Obstructive shock**, eg cardiac tamponade.

6   OXYGEN DELIVERY

How can oxygen be delivered to a patient?

Variable performance devices:

- Nasal cannulae
- Face mask – at 2 litres/minute, approximate $Fio_2 = 0.25$–0.30; at 6–10 litres/minute, $Fio_2 = 0.30$–0.40.

Fixed performance devices (constant Fio_2):

- Venturi mask – nozzle designed to entrain air with oxygen; affords specific Fio_2 depending on nozzle used
- Reservoir bag – Fio_2 close to 1.0; mostly used in trauma
- Continuous positive airway pressure (CPAP)
- Invasive ventilatory support.

What is the danger of oxygen therapy in a patient who has chronic carbon dioxide retention?

- Uncontrolled use of oxygen may cause apnoea.
- Some patients with chronically raised carbon dioxide rely on hypoxia to stimulate respiration. If this drive is abolished through the use of high concentrations of oxygen, this can lead to apnoea.
- Correction of hypoxia may reverse the normal compensatory hypoxic venoconstriction, leading to worsening $\dot{V}/\dot{Q}$ mismatch.

What are the potential complications of oxygen therapy?

- **Absorption atelectasis** – nitrogen is slowly absorbed and therefore splints the alveoli; high concentrations of oxygen flush out the nitrogen. Oxygen is absorbed rapidly and the alveoli collapse.
- **Pulmonary toxicity** – oxygen irritates the mucosa of the airways directly, leading to loss of surfactant and progressive fibrosis.
- **Retinopathy** due to retrolenticular fibroplasia.
- **Risk of fires and explosions**.

7   PULMONARY ARTERY WEDGE CATHETER

What can a pulmonary artery wedge catheter (PAWC) measure, and what can it be used for?

It is a 70–80-cm long catheter with 10-cm markings. It usually has three to four lumens:

- Distal
- Proximal
- Injectate
- Lumen for balloon inflation.

Indications:

- Optimisation of fluid therapy (especially if right atrial pressures do not reflect left heart function, as in severe bundle branch block, pulmonary hypertension, tamponade or pericarditis)
- Rationalisation of inotropic support
- Investigation of cardiac shunts
- Measurement of cardiac output.

How do you insert a PAWC?

- Insert in the same fashion as a central venous pressure line.
- Use aseptic Seldinger technique, with continuous visible pressure monitoring.
- Correct positioning confirmed by pressure changes as PAWC is advanced (central venous pressure, atrial, right ventricle and, finally, pulmonary artery pressures).
- 'Wedge' pressure achieved when balloon occludes pulmonary vessel, so creating a continuous column of blood to left atrium.

What measurements can be made using a PAWC?

Direct measurements:

- Mixed venous gases
- Pulmonary artery pressures
- Right atrial and ventricular pressures
- Right ventricular ejection fraction
- Right cardiac output.

Indirect measurements:

- Systemic vascular resistance
- Peripheral vascular resistance
- Cardiac index (CI)
- Stroke volume index.

Note that the usual pulmonary artery pressure is approximately a fifth of the systemic pressure (15–30 mmHg systolic, 0–8 mmHg diastolic, mean 10–15 mmHg).

8   ARTIFICIAL VENTILATION

What are the indications for artificial ventilation?

- Respiratory failure (respiratory rate >30 breaths/minute, high $PaCO_2$), exhaustion
- Head injury/coma (to reduce intracranial pressure)
- Severe shock
- Loss of chest wall integrity (trauma)
- Peripheral neuromuscular disease (Guillain–Barré syndrome)
- To reduce the work of breathing, eg in cardiac failure.

What are the complications of artificial ventilation?

- Cardiovascular complications:
  - decrease in venous return
  - increase in pulmonary vascular resistance, leading to decreased right and left ventricular output
- Ventilatory trauma – barotrauma leading to pneumothorax
- Nosocomial infection (atelectasis)
- ARDS
- Water retention (release of vasopressin)
- Respiratory muscle wasting.

What are the indications for tracheostomy?

- Surgical access
- Relief of airway obstruction
- Protection of tracheobronchial tree
- Suction and removal of secretions
- Prolonged ventilation (>10–14 days, slow to wean off).

9   NUTRITIONAL SUPPORT

What are the basic components of total parenteral nutrition (TPN)?

Water, potassium, sodium, energy, nitrogen, magnesium, phosphate, water-soluble vitamins, trace elements and essential fatty acids.

What are the complications of TPN?

- **Catheter-related:**
  - insertion
  - displacement
  - infection
  - thrombosis
  - occlusion
- **Metabolic:**
  - hyper/hypoglycaemia
  - hyper/hypokalaemia
  - hypophosphataemia
  - metabolic acidosis
- **Fluid overload**
- **Deficiencies of vitamins and trace elements**
- **Hepatobiliary:**
  - abnormal liver function tests
  - jaundice
- **Intestinal:**
  - villous atrophy
  - bacterial translocation/endotoxaemia.

What are the indications for nutritional support?

- Patients who are unable to maintain adequate nutrition to maintain body haemostasis
- Medical and surgical disorders likely to result in malnutrition, eg intestinal fistulae, Crohn's disease
- Postoperative starvation lasting more than 10 days.

10 ITU VERSUS HDU

Which patients should be admitted to an HDU (High Dependency Unit)?

Patients for admission to HDU are typically those who need a higher level of monitoring and/or nursing than is available on a general ward but who do not need ventilation:

- High-risk surgical patients (with medical co-morbidities), for monitoring/support
- Patients who have undergone major/complex surgical procedures, eg hepatic resection, oesophagectomy
- Patients at risk of developing multiple-organ failure/ dysfunction, eg pancreatitis
- Patients able to step down from ITU care.

What are the selection criteria for admitting a patient to an ITU (Intensive Therapy Unit)?

- Major organ failure – patients requiring artificial support (respiratory, cardiovascular, etc)
- Severe disease states in which intensive monitoring and treatment is required (septicaemia, head injury, etc.)
- Homeostatic disorders (severe fluid and electrolyte imbalance, thermoregulatory failure)
- Patients who are undergoing specialised therapeutic techniques and/or monitoring.

What is 'multiple-organ failure' (MOF)?

- A syndrome characterised by the significant failure of two or more organs.
- Usually starts with minor or moderate abnormalities in organ function (multiple-organ dysfunction syndrome, or MODS). Failure to control the situation at this stage may lead to MOF.
- Five main organ systems (with various definitions for specific organ system failure):
  - cardiovascular
  - respiratory
  - renal
  - haematological
  - neurological.
- Additional features include:
  - polyneuropathy
  - gastrointestinal failure (ileus)
  - musculoskeletal failure (muscle wasting, myositis)
  - skin 'failure' (pressure sores)
  - endocrine failure (hypoadrenalism, abnormal thyroid function tests).

11   INOTROPIC SUPPORT

What different inotropic agents are available?

- Catecholamines (adrenaline (epinephrine), noradrenaline (norepinephrine), dobutamine, dopamine)
- Phosphodiesterase inhibitors (enoximone, milrinone)
- Calcium
- Glucagon (possibly via increased calcium influx)
- Cardiac glycosides (digoxin – weak, hardly used).

What are their modes of action and common side effects?

- β1-agonists increase the force of myocardial contraction.
- Phosphodiesterase inhibitors decrease cAMP breakdown, increasing contractility.
- Side effects:
  - arrhythmia
  - tachycardia
  - hypertension
  - exacerbation of ischaemia (ECG changes occur due to increased oxygen demand)
  - hyperglycaemia.

When would you consider initiating inotropic support on ITU?

The choice of inotrope depends on the clinical circumstances:

- Low cardiac output states, eg ventricular dysfunction – consider adrenaline, enoximone or dobutamine
- Vasodilatation, eg sepsis – use noradrenaline
- Raised pulmonary vascular resistance – use enoximone.

12   INFECTION ON ITU

What clinical findings on ITU would lead you to suspect that a patient is harbouring an infection?

- Pyrexia
- Elevated white cell count
- Altered neurological state
- Cardiovascular instability
- Productive cough (or increased secretions on suction)
- Changes on chest X-ray
- Rising platelet count
- Persistently low albumin.

What factors increase the risk of infection?

Pre-hospital factors:

- Extremes of age
- Underlying disease, eg diabetes
- Malnutrition
- Immunosuppression
- Lifestyle, eg smoking.

Intra-hospital factors:

- Underlying disease on admission to ITU, eg aspiration
- Organ failure, eg renal failure
- Damage to skin/mucosal surfaces
- Surgery
- Prolonged hospitalisation.

ITU factors:

- Poor adherence to hygiene protocols
- Reduced bed space
- Reduced staffing levels
- Contaminated airflow/equipment
- Invasive procedures
- Mechanical ventilation
- Catheterisation
- Antibiotics.

How would you attempt to control infection on ITU?

- Use of plastic aprons when approaching patients
- Hand-washing techniques
- Single-patient nursing
- Single-patient equipment
- Isolation of infected patients (cubicles)
- Staff education
- Use of aseptic technique for invasive procedures
- Early identification of infections and targeted antimicrobial therapy
- Minimisation of potential infection routes (eg removal of arterial or venous lines that are no longer needed).

13   HEAD INJURIES

How do you assess the severity of a head injury?

- Glasgow Coma Scale (GCS):

13–15	Minor
9–12	Moderate
3–8	Severe

- Observation of pupil size (unequal pupils)
- Bradycardia and hypertension – may suggest raised intracranial pressure (although this may be masked in trauma)
- Unequal motor response
- Imaging – skull and cervical spine X-rays, CT scan of head.

How would you manage a severe head injury?

- Advanced Trauma Life Support (ATLS) guidelines (ABCDE)
- GCS score less than 9 warrants consideration of intubation/ventilation
- Also consider transfer to specialist centre.

How would you manage a severe head injury on ITU?

- General – avoid hypoxia, hypotension, hypoperfusion (with supportive treatment, eg ventilation, inotropes)
- Reduce raised intracranial pressure if feasible – hyperventilation (only short-term), diuretics (mannitol), sedation, mild hypothermia
- Suspect cervical spine injury
- Keep blood sugar within normal limits
- Keep plasma osmolality between 310 mosmol/kg and 320 mosmol/kg
- Use anticonvulsants if seizure activity is likely
- Other measures:
    - nutrition
    - antibiotics.

14   BRAINSTEM DEATH

What are structures in the brainstem?

- Midbrain
- Pons
- Medulla oblongata.

These contain:

- Respiratory and cardiovascular centres
- Reticular activating system (a diffuse area of the upper brainstem, necessary for consciousness)
- Areas for integration of sensory and motor traffic from the cranial nerves.

What conditions must be met before a diagnosis of brainstem death can be made?

General:

- Irremediable brain damage
- Exclusion of reversible causes for absent brainstem function
- Comatose patient/ventilated
- Known aetiology for the coma.

Exclusion of:

- Hypothermia
- Metabolic/endocrine disturbance
- Depression of central nervous system due to drugs
- Recent circulatory arrest.

How would you determine brainstem death?

These tests should be performed by at least two doctors, of whom at least one is a consultant, and should be repeated:

- No pupillary response to light (IInd cranial nerve)
- Absent corneal blink reflex (Vth and VIIth cranial nerves)
- No occulovestibular reflex (IIIrd and VIth cranial nerves): tested using cold stimulation of tympanic membrane, after confirmation of clear auditory canal – this stimulus should provoke no response (normal response is deviation towards syringed ear)
- No motor response in the distribution of the cranial nerves (no grimacing)
- No gag or cough reflex on tracheal/bronchial stimulation
- No ventilatory effort following apnoeic test (P_{CO_2} has to rise to 6.65 kPa) – after disconnection from ventilator.

15   SEDATION ON ITU

What are the most common indications for sedation on ITU?

- Mechanical ventilation
- Invasive procedures
- Pain/discomfort
- Underlying medical conditions:
  - raised intracranial pressure
  - seizures
  - low cardiac output state.

What are the undesirable effects of sedation?

- Inability to fully evaluate the patient's neurological status
- Cardiovascular instability
- More intravenous access required (therefore greater risk of infection)
- Decreased clearance of the drugs used for sedation may prolong weaning from ventilatory support.

Which sedative drugs are used on the ITU?

- Benzodiazepines – midazolam
- Intravenous anaesthetic agents – propofol
- Barbiturates – thiopentone in status epilepticus
- Inhalational anaesthetic agents – isoflurane.

16   RENAL FAILURE

What do you understand by the term 'prerenal failure' and what are the causes of this condition?

- Inadequate renal perfusion due to reduced intravascular volume or lowered effective arterial circulation.
- Commonest surgical causes include:
  - gastrointestinal losses
  - haemorrhage
  - sepsis
  - third-space losses (eg pancreatitis).
- May lead to acute tubular necrosis if untreated.

What are the other causes of renal failure and how may they be classified?

Prerenal:

- Renal artery disease
- Abdominal aortic aneurysm
- Malignant hypertension.

Renal:

- Acute tubular necrosis
- Glomerulonephritis
- Drugs.

Postrenal:

- Bilateral ureteric obstruction
- Calculus in a solitary kidney.

How may examination of the urine be useful in the management of acute renal failure?

- The presence of white cells suggests infection or inflammation.
- Haematuria suggests stones or tumour.
- Whole casts suggests intrinsic disease (eg glomerulonephritis).
- Protein suggests glomerular injury.
- Specific gravity >1.022 suggests intact concentrating ability.
- Spot urinary sodium concentration may help differentiate prerenal failure from acute tubular necrosis (fractional sodium excretion in prerenal failure is <1%; fractional sodium excretion in acute tubular necrosis is >1%).
- Urine culture for infection.

17   CARDIAC OUTPUT

Which clinical parameters can be used to estimate cardiac output?

- Conscious level
- Blood pressure
- Pulse pressure
- Heart rate
- Temperature
- Urine output
- Peripheral perfusion
- Capillary refill.

How do you measure cardiac output?

Fick principle:

- Requires samples of mixed venous and arterial blood.
- Cardiac output (litres/minute):

$$\frac{O_2 \text{ absorbed per minute by lungs (ml/min)}}{\text{Arteriovenous } O_2 \text{ difference (ml/l of blood)}}$$

Dilution technique:

- **Dye dilution** – known amount of dye is injected and its concentration measured peripherally (photoelectric spectrometer), indocyanine green (low half-life and toxicity)
- **Thermodilution** – uses cold saline, data represented as temperature drop against time; cardiac output is inversely proportional to the area under the curve.

Are you aware of any other methods of measuring cardiac output?

- Impedance plethysmography
- Echocardiography
- Electromagnetic flow measurement (probe on aortic root during surgery)
- Cardiac catheterisation
- Oesophageal Doppler.

18   RESPIRATORY FAILURE

Define respiratory failure and what are its clinical signs?

PaO_2 less than 8 kPa while breathing air without intracardiac shunting.

Signs:

- Cyanosis
- Tachypnoea
- Use of accessory muscles
- Inability to speak in sentences
- Depressed level of consciousness
- Signs of hypercapnia.

What is the difference between type 1 and type 2 respiratory failure?

Type 1 respiratory failure:

- Low Po_2 with normal or low Pco_2, usually due to $\dot{V}/\dot{Q}$ mismatch (eg chest infection, pulmonary oedema, pulmonary embolism, ARDS, aspiration pneumonitis)
- Pco_2 low in response to increased respiratory effort (low Po_2).

Type 2 respiratory failure:

- Low Po_2 with high Pco_2, usually due to ventilatory failure (eg exacerbation of COPD, end-stage asthma).

How can you treat respiratory failure?

- Treat underlying cause
- Oxygen
- Respiratory stimulants, eg doxapram
- Continuous positive airway pressure (CPAP)
- Intermittent positive-pressure ventilation (IPPV)
- Extracorporeal membrane oxygenation (ECMO).

19   PULSE OXIMETRY

What information can be gained from pulse oximetry?

- Oxygen saturation (SaO_2) of haemoglobin
- Pulse rate
- Peripheral perfusion.

What factors might make pulse oximetry unreliable?

- Patient movement
- Electrical interference (diathermy)
- Venous congestion
- SaO_2 below 50%
- Coloured nail polish
- Carboxyhaemoglobin (SaO_2 falsely high)
- Methaemoglobin, bilirubin (SaO_2 falsely low)
- Methylene blue dye (decreases SaO_2 temporarily)
- Ambient light.

Note that fetal haemoglobin (HbF) and polycythaemia have no effect on readings.

How does pulse oximetry work?

- Pulse oximetry relies on the principle that absorbance of light by a substance depends on the concentration of the substance and the distance the light travels through it (Beer–Lambert law).
- Two light-emitting diodes produce beams at red and near infrared frequencies (660 nm and 980 nm), which are picked up by a photodetector on the opposite side.
- Diodes flash approximately 30 times per second.
- A microprocessor analyses light absorption during arterial flow and ignores non-pulsatile components of the signal (tissues and venous blood).

20   PREOPERATIVE RESPIRATORY ASSESSMENT

How would you assess a patient with severe respiratory disease for surgery?

History:

- Previous admissions or ITU care
- Exercise tolerance
- Cough
- Home oxygen
- Smoking.

Examination:

- Cyanosis
- Dyspnoea at rest
- Chest auscultation and percussion for active disease.

What investigations would you perform?

- Spirometry:
  - peak expiratory flow rate
  - FEV_1
  - FVC
  - FEV_1/FVC ratio
- Arterial blood gases
- Flow–volume loops
- Chest X-ray
- CT thorax (if indicated).

How would you identify a high-risk respiratory patient?

- FEV_1 <1000 ml
- FEV_1/FVC <50%
- Pa_{CO_2} >6 kPa
- Body mass index (BMI) >27 kg/m^2
- Peak flow <200 litres/minute
- Age >60 years.

21   CENTRAL VENOUS PRESSURE

What are the indications for gaining central venous access?

- Vascular access
- Measurement of central venous pressure (CVP)
- Insertion of pulmonary artery wedge catheter
- Transvenous pacing
- Parenteral feeding (long-term).

What problems can be associated with central venous access?

- Infection
- Arrhythmias
- Air embolism
- Cardiac/lung perforation
- Central vein thrombosis
- Neurovascular damage.

What are the components of the venous waveform?

a wave – atrial contraction.
c wave – tricuspid valve bulges back into the atrium during ventricular isometric systolic phase.
x descent – atrial relaxation.
v wave – rise in atrial pressure before the tricuspid valve opens.
y descent – atrial emptying into the ventricle.

Notes:

- No *a* wave in atrial fibrillation
- Enlarged *a* wave in tricuspid stenosis, pulmonary hypertension
- Enlarged *v* wave in tricuspid regurgitation
- Cannon waves (not corresponding to *a*, *v*, or *c* waves) in:
  - complete heart block (irregular)
  - junctional arrhythmias (regular).

22   PRESSURE SORES

What is a pressure sore?

- A term used to describe a range of destructive lesions of the skin and subcutaneous tissues which are of varied pathogenesis.
- Also referred to as 'bed sores', 'decubitus ulcers', 'pressure ulcers' and 'brush burns'.
- Range in severity from erythematous soft-tissue lesions to open wounds which extend deep into the tissues.

Which patients are at risk from pressure sores?

Waterlow pressure sore risk factors:

- High BMI
- Incontinence
- Frail skin
- Immobility (sedated, bed-bound, neurological deficit)
- Poor tissue nutrition (cachexia, cardiac failure, peripheral vascular disease, anaemia, smoking)
- Major surgery/trauma
- Poor appetite
- Elderly
- Immunosuppressant medication (cytotoxics, high-dose steroids, anti-inflammatories).

How can pressure sores be prevented?

- Identify at-risk individuals (on admission).
- Have a policy for nursing staff for pressure care nursing (turning, padding, mattresses).
- Skin condition should be inspected daily (especially bony prominences) with reassessment of risk.
- Frequent repositioning, eg avoid sitting in chair for more than 2 hours.
- Find and eliminate any sources of excess moisture, eg due to incontinence, perspiration or wound drainage.
- Nutritional support.
- Early mobilisation.

23   CARDIOPULMONARY BYPASS

What are the indications for cardiopulmonary bypass?

- Cardiothoracic surgery:
  - coronary revascularisation
  - cardiac valvular surgery
  - surgery on the thoracic aorta
- Neurosurgery, eg for basilar artery aneurysm
- Supportive treatment of critically ill patients, eg severe hypothermia, drug overdose.

What are the components of a cardiopulmonary bypass system?

Blood is drained from the superior and inferior vena cavae by gravity into a venous reservoir, which is then passed through an oxygenator and a heat exchanger. This arterialised blood is returned via a bubble trap and microemboli filter through the aortic cannula to the systemic circulation. Blood is also returned from suction systems and cardiac vents, through a microfilter, into the circulation.

What are the complications of cardiopulmonary bypass?

There may be complications during cardiopulmonary bypass and complications may also arise in the early and late phases after bypass.

Complications during cardiopulmonary bypass:

- Disruption of the circuit – massive air embolism, hypoxia from pump failure, venous congestion from misplaced or kinked lines
- Coagulopathy and hypersensitivity reactions to heparin
- Inflammatory response resulting from contact of blood with non-endothelial circuit surfaces
- Anaemia from haemodilution and red cell damage from pump
- Hypothermia.

Early post-bypass complications:

- Cardiac arrhythmias (atrial and ventricular)
- Pulmonary (atelectasis, ARDS)
- Acute renal failure (uncommon).

Late post-bypass complications:

- Focal neurological deficits (may be temporary or permanent)
- Seizures
- Coma/stupor
- Respiratory injury
- Mesenteric ischaemia
- Pancreatitis.

24   SCORING SYSTEMS ON ITU

In general, what types of illness scoring are used in the critical care setting?

1   Scores to estimate patient outcome and to guide clinical management.

2   Scores to stratify patients for audit and research purposes.

Can you give some examples of each type?

1   Scores to estimate patient outcome and to guide clinical management:
- RTS – **R**evised **T**rauma **S**core
- ISS – **I**njury **S**everity **S**core
- MEWS – **M**odified **E**arly **W**arning **S**ystem.

2   Scores to stratify patients for audit and research purposes:
- APACHE II score – **A**cute **P**hysiology **A**nd **C**hronic **H**ealth status **E**valuation
- POSSUM – **P**hysiological and **O**perative **S**everity **S**core for the en**UM**eration of morbidity and mortality.

What are the limitations of ITU scoring systems?

- Intra- and interobserver error
- Accuracy of data
- Insufficient data
- Systems such as the ISS require data that may not all be available early on in the clinical course
- Over-reliance on scores rather than clinical judgement.

25   SYSTEMIC INFLAMMATORY RESPONSE SYNDROME

What is the difference between systemic inflammatory response syndrome (SIRS), sepsis and septic shock?

SIRS is defined by the presence of two of the following criteria:

- Temperature >38.4 °C or <35.6 °C
- Heart rate >90 bpm
- Respiratory rate >40 breaths/minute, or P_{CO_2} <32 mmHg (4.2 kPa)
- White cell count >12,000/ml, <4,000/ml, or >10% immature forms.

Sepsis is SIRS with documented infection.

Septic shock is sepsis with tissue hypoperfusion.

What are the causes of SIRS?

SIRS is the response of the body to an infectious or non-infectious insult. Infectious insults are more common and are usually due to Gram-negative bacteria, but this also occurs in response to infections with viruses, other bacteria, fungi and higher organisms. Non-infectious causes include trauma, burns and pancreatitis.

What mediators are involved in SIRS?

- There are bacterial factors and host factors.
- Bacterial cell walls (endotoxin) and various exotoxins, such as toxic shock syndrome toxin-1, act directly on immune cells to activate the inflammatory response.
- In response to the inflammatory stimulus, host cells release pro-inflammatory cytokines such as interleukin 1 (IL-1), interleukin 6 (IL-6) and tumour necrosis factor-α (TNF-α). These are kept in check by anti-inflammatory cytokines such as interleukin 10 (IL-10) and transforming growth factor-β (TGF-β).
- The balance of the pro-inflammatory and anti-inflammatory factors determines the response.

26 JAUNDICE

What is bilirubin and how is it metabolised?

- Bilirubin is a pigment and metabolic end-product of haem degradation. Most bilirubin is derived from the breakdown of senescent red blood cells, with approximately 20% from other haem-containing proteins, such as myoglobin and the cytochrome complexes.
- Haem is degraded by haem oxygenase to biliverdin, which is reduced to bilirubin.
- Bilirubin is insoluble and is strongly bound to albumin in plasma, where it is transported to the liver. Here, it is taken up by active transport into the hepatocytes and conjugated to glucuronic acid, rendering it water-soluble.
- The conjugated bilirubins are secreted into bile and enter the gut.
- Some of the conjugated bilirubins are broken down into urobilinogen by gut bacteria, which is freely permeable through the bowel wall, and enters the circulation to be excreted in the urine.
- The rest of the bilirubin enters the colon where it is converted to stercobilinogens by the gut bacteria and excreted in faeces.
- A fraction of the stercobilinogen and urobilinogens are reabsorbed into the enterohepatic circulation.

How is jaundice classified?

- **Prehepatic** – due to increased production of bilirubin, beyond the capacity of hepatic conjugation, eg haemolytic anaemia
- **Hepatic** – due to impaired uptake or conjugation of bilirubin as a result of hepatocellular dysfunction, eg hepatitis, Gilbert's syndrome
- **Post-hepatic** – due to obstruction of the biliary tree, preventing the elimination of conjugated bilirubin, eg gallstones and carcinoma of the head of pancreas.

What are the important aspects of perioperative care in the jaundiced patient?

- Coagulopathy due to impaired vitamin K absorption
- Development of hepatorenal syndrome – keep patients adequately hydrated
- Development of drug toxicity due to impaired hepatic metabolism.

27 VALVULAR HEART DISEASE

Which patients are at risk of endocarditis and what precautions should be taken in these patients?

Patients at risk of endocarditis are those with:

- Heart valve lesions
- Septal defects
- Patent ductus arteriosus
- Prosthetic heart valves
- Previous history of endocarditis.

Invasive procedures have the potential to cause transient bacteraemia, including dental procedures, genitourinary procedures, gastrointestinal procedures, upper respiratory tract procedures and obstetric and gynaecological procedures. Prophylactic antibiotics should be administered pre- and post-procedure.

What are the salient points in the perioperative management of patients with aortic stenosis?

- Aortic stenosis causes left ventricular outflow obstruction and eventually a fixed low-output state which is associated with high mortality. These patients are at high risk of major perioperative cardiac events, including myocardial infarction, arrhythmias and sudden cardiac death.
- Perioperative management should include a careful assessment of cardiac and valvular function, most easily achieved by echocardiography.
- In the event of severe valvular stenosis, the patient should be considered for valve surgery prior to other procedures.
- Other disturbances which compromise cardiac function, such as atrial fibrillation, should be corrected or optimised.
- At induction, antibiotics should be given for endocarditis prophylaxis.
- The anaesthetic is selected in order to maintain haemodynamic stability and, in particular, any manoeuvres which lower systemic vascular resistance must be avoided.
- Postoperatively, the patient should be monitored closely, watching for the development of complications such as cardiac failure and infarction.

What are the complications of prosthetic cardiac valves?

Early complications:

- Structural damage during valve insertion – damage to the coronary circulation, conduction system or cardiac rupture

- Complications arising from the use of cardiopulmonary bypass, including bleeding and anaemia.

Late complications:

- Thrombosis
- Infection
- Valve failure – can result from degeneration of the valve from calcification, ingrowth of pannus, mechanical failure (such as strut fractures in the old valves)
- Embolisation of valve fragments
- Valve dehiscence and paravalvular leaks related to the surgical technique or infection.

28   CARDIAC ARREST

How would you assess a collapsed and unresponsive patient on the ward?

- Check the patient's responsiveness – 'shake and shout'.
- Open the airway – head tilt/jaw lift.
- Check the respiratory effort – look, listen and feel.
- If not breathing and unresponsive, make five attempts to give two full effective breaths using a face mask.
- Call for help – ask someone to put out an adult cardiac arrest call via the switchboard.
- Assess the circulation for 10 seconds at the carotid.
- If circulation present, continue artificial respiration.
- If circulation not present, commence chest compressions at a ratio of 15 compressions to every two breaths.

How would you classify the reversible causes of cardiac arrest?

The four 'T's and the four 'H's:

- **T**ension pneumothorax
- **T**amponade (cardiac)
- **T**oxic/therapeutic disturbances
- **T**hromboembolic
- **H**ypothermia
- **H**yper/hypokalaemia
- **H**ypoxia
- **H**ypovolaemia.

How would you treat a right-sided tension pneumothorax?

The diagnosis of a right-sided tension pneumothorax is made by the presence of signs of circulatory embarrassment, tachypnoea, hyper-resonance to percussion, reduced breath sounds and deviation of the trachea away from the side of the tension pneumothorax.

- Tension pneumothorax is an emergency and should be treated immediately with the insertion of a large-bore cannula into the second right intercostal space in the mid-clavicular line. This decompresses the tension but a formal chest tube is needed.
- The chest tube should be placed just anterior to the mid-axillary line in the fifth intercostal space.
- It should be performed using an aseptic technique with Betadine® skin preparation and infiltration of local anaesthesia.
- An incision is made above the rib, with blunt dissection with artery forceps down to the pleura.
- Once the pleura is breached, a finger is inserted and any lung tissue is swept away.

- The chest tube is inserted (after discarding the trocar) with the aid of a pair of artery forceps and the tube is positioned appropriately.
- The tube is then secured with a silk suture, dressed and attached to an underwater seal drainage system.

29   FAT EMBOLISM

What is an embolus?

An embolus is an abnormal collection of undissolved matter that traverses the vascular system from one point to another. It is commonly a thrombus, but it may be gas (eg air or nitrogen), solid (eg tumour cells, foreign body) or liquid (fat, amniotic fluid).

How does fat embolism occur?

Fat embolism usually occurs after a closed fracture of a long bone, in severe trauma without a fracture, or in severe non-traumatic illness. It is thought to occur via two mechanisms:

1   The **mechanical theory** postulates that fat droplets gain entry to the circulation through the damaged vasculature at the fracture site (although this does not explain the non-traumatic causes).
2   The **metabolic theory** postulates that there is release and activation of lipases within the circulation, liberating free fatty acids and glycerol (and also 5-hydroxytryptamine from platelets, leading to bronchospasm).

What is the clinical picture in fat embolism and how is it treated?

The diagnosis of fat embolism requires a high index of clinical suspicion. The petechial rash over the chest, axilla, mouth and conjunctivae is pathognomonic, and the presence of lipid in the mucus and urine is highly specific.

There is a triad of **clinical signs**:

- Petechial rash
- Respiratory insufficiency – tachypnoea and cyanosis; due to V/Q mismatch, pneumonitis, superadded pneumonia or ARDS
- Cerebral features – in 90%, often the earliest sign; commonly encephalopathy (due to microembolisation to cerebral vessels and/or lipase-mediated cerebral damage).

Non-specific signs include pyrexia, tachycardia, retinopathy and renal impairment.

Treatment is firstly supportive, with:

- Oxygen therapy – CPAP or IPPV
- Fluid and electrolyte monitoring
- Prophylaxis of DVT, pneumonia
- Nutritional and skin care.

Specific therapies include:

- Corticosteroids
- Albumin
- Intravenous ethanol
- Heparin.

The clinical benefit of these specific treatments has not yet been proved.

30   CARE OF THE MULTIPLY INJURED

A patient is brought to the Emergency Department after a road traffic accident with burns to his chest and arms, an obviously fractured femur and signs of a base of skull fracture. Describe the first stages of your management.

Follow the **ATLS guidelines** in initiating a primary survey. Do not move on to the next step before all uncovered pathologies have been stabilised. Return to reassess if the condition changes during the survey.

Primary survey:

- **Airway** with cervical spine control – note if the patient is talking and, if not, whether they are spontaneously maintaining an airway.
- **Breathing** – assess bilateral air entry, respiratory rate, character and depth, and monitor oxygenation with a saturation probe.
- **Circulation** with haemorrhage control – assess carotid pulse rate and take a blood pressure reading while gaining intravenous access (take bloods, including a glucose measurement, and start an intravenous infusion of Hartmann's solution).
- **Disability** – assess the patient's neurological function and calculate their Glasgow Coma Scale (GCS) score.
- **Exposure** with environmental control.
- Order a trauma series of X-rays (chest X-ray, pelvis and lateral cervical spine views) before any further intervention.

Move on to the **secondary survey**, with examination from skull to toes for injuries.

Can you describe the specific management required for the femoral fracture, chest burns and head injury?

Each of the injuries will have been appropriately stabilised at the time of the primary survey.

The **head injury** should be assessed as mentioned and if there are signs of base of skull fracture (decreased GCS, rhinorrhoea, otorrhoea, haemotympanum or periorbital haematomas) or indeed just a decrease in GCS with this history of head trauma, then a CT scan should be obtained once the patient has been stabilised.

The **burns** should be treated according to their extent and depth and the fluid balance must be attended to. Fluid replacement can be calculated using a number of formulae, such as the Parkland formula or the Muir and Barclay formula. Consider an escharotomy if respiratory function is compromised. Definitive care should be discussed with the regional burns unit.

The **femoral shaft fracture** should be assessed, reduced and stabilised with in-line traction to reduce the possibility of neurovascular compromise distally, pain, and fat embolus. A patient with an open fracture will require intravenous antibiotics and a Betadine®-soaked dressing. X-rays should be taken to plan the orthopaedic management.

What is the trimodal distribution of death in trauma?

There are three peaks in the incidence of death due to trauma:

- Immediate deaths, due to massive head and thoracic injuries
- Secondary peak, after minutes to hours, due to subdural haematomas, hypoxia and hypovolaemia
- A late peak, after days to weeks, due to sepsis and multiple-organ failure.

7

COMMUNICATION SKILLS

How to approach communication skills

HOW TO APPROACH COMMUNICATION SKILLS

The objectives of communication skills testing are:

- To assess the ability of the candidate to assimilate and understand medical facts in a short space of time (ie information gathering).
- To determine how good the candidate is at presenting information to a patient in language that they will understand (ie information giving).
- To test the candidate by presenting 'difficult' scenarios that may be very taxing to resolve.

It is usual practice for actors to replace patients and they are generally briefed thoroughly and carefully – they will know the scenario much better than you will!

Preparation

Read the case through carefully and make sure you know how long you have to prepare the case before being called into the examination. Remember to take paper and pens with you (if allowed), to make notes and to ensure that the scenario is clear in your mind. The following are general points to consider:

1   Am I supposed to know this patient/relative?
2   Is he or she someone I see every day on the ward round?
3   Is this a relative who has just arrived from out of town to talk to me?
4   Which area of the hospital am I in (eg Outpatients Department, ITU)?
5   Classify the problems into medical, social and psychological – deal with each of these separately.
6   'Edit' the case to remove extraneous information. For example, there may be a list of blood results, most of which are entirely irrelevant to the task.
7   What is the patient's frame of mind likely to be? Are they angry, depressed or bereaved? This is best assessed by asking yourself the question, 'How would I feel if . . . ?'
8   Make a plan for your conversation.

During the scenario

The following tips are useful for the exam:

- Points are awarded for the approach to the actor or patient and you should either introduce yourself formally (if you have never met the patient before) or remind the patient who you are (eg if you have met frequently on ward rounds).

- You should draw a diagram to illustrate a point if necessary.
- Never talk down to the patient.
- Avoid any medical jargon (such as 'history' or 'neoplasm').
- Remember that you must attempt to complete the task. If you are asked to obtain consent for organ donation, for example, you must be seen to be making an effort to achieve this or you may not pass.
- You also may not pass if the medical information you provide is entirely inaccurate, although you are not being formally assessed on your surgical knowledge in this part of the exam.
- Finally, be aware that the actor may well have an input into the marks you are awarded for the case.

1   DEALING WITH ANGRY PATIENTS OR RELATIVES

Scenario

You are a Specialist Registrar in the Emergency Department.

At the end of an 11-hour shift, you have picked up your last card from the 'waiting to be seen' box. A 34-year-old solicitor has brought her 7-year-old daughter back to the department this evening. She was seen by one of your colleagues this morning and discharged home with a 'stomach bug'. Now the girl is tachycardic, pyrexial and showing signs of peritonitis. She has been transferred to the care of the paediatricians to be resuscitated prior to undergoing a laparotomy for suspected ruptured appendicitis.

Her mother has had to cancel a crucial meeting with a legal client (which would have generated a £50,000 contract) in order to return to the department and is devastated that her daughter has become so critically ill during the day. The Consultant is at home and there are no seniors immediately available. You have to explain to the mother what has happened and why her daughter requires urgent surgery.

Preparation – things to consider

Reading the scenario, it is clear that the communication skill being tested here is your ability to 'deal with' an angry patient or, in this case, an angry relative. This is extremely difficult and must be thought out carefully. There are certain 'hooks' which your consultation should be based on, in order to underpin a successful outcome:

- Encourage the relative to sit down somewhere quiet with you rather than conduct a shouting match in a very public area.
- Avoid covering up for colleagues who made, in retrospect, an incorrect diagnosis.
- Avoid blaming anyone for what has happened.
- Apologise to the relative but do not take personal blame for the incident.

Approach

Begin by introducing yourself – the mother has met a lot of different doctors during the day and it is important that she realises that you are not the surgeon or paediatrician, but the Casualty Officer. The various aspects of the scenario can be broken down into medical, social and psychological issues.

Medical

- Unfortunately you are responsible in her eyes for your colleague's earlier error.

- Ask her to sit down if she is pacing about, and explain what has happened.
- Give her a chance to vent her fury before trying to interject.
- Do not second-guess what happened at the earlier consultation – **you were not there** and therefore cannot possibly know what your colleague said.
- Try to move the discussion on to focus on her daughter, aligning yourself with her maternal concern and telling her repeatedly that the teams are working in her daughter's best interests.

Social

- The scenario does not make it clear whether there are other children at home or who else is at home with the family. You should ask if there is anyone else at home to be taken care of – this is something you may be able to organise in order to alleviate any further problems (eg by contacting a neighbour to help).

Psychological

- Be understanding – put yourself into this lady's shoes.
- Expect that she will be angry, even unreasonable, but your reaction would be the same in similar circumstances – remember that she has a critically ill daughter, she has presumably lost a legal contract and she is looking for someone to blame.
- She may feel guilty that she did not return her daughter to hospital earlier.
- A successful outcome in this case depends on your ability to empathise with this mother, sharing her concerns, sadness and sympathy (but not her **anger**).
- You must not come across as combative or awkward but, equally, do not fall into the trap of condemning or criticising your colleague's earlier actions.

Minimum requirements

- You must attempt to stop her shouting (if she is) by the end of your time with her.
- You must show empathy and be sympathetic to her feelings.
- You must not criticise your colleague's earlier actions.
- Explain who she must speak to next, so that she is kept fully informed of her daughter's progress.

2   BREAKING BAD NEWS

Scenario

The patient is a 64-year-old retired music teacher who recently presented to the Emergency Department with a 3-month history of lethargy, tiredness and loss of appetite. She had been forced to come to the hospital by a worried neighbour. She was widowed 2 years ago and has a daughter who lives in South Africa. You examined her originally and palpated a mass in the right iliac fossa. She had a microcytic anaemia at that time and she was subsequently transfused. She had a barium enema today, which she found very uncomfortable, and you have just reviewed the films with the radiologist – these show an apple-core lesion in the right side of the colon. An ultrasound examination of the abdomen was normal. Your Consultant has scheduled her for tomorrow's operating list.

You are the Senior House Officer on the firm and the Consultant is planning to return to the ward tomorrow to obtain her consent for surgery. You have been asked to explain the results of the tests to her.

Preparation – things to consider

- You have met this lady before, so the way to begin is to ask her what she already knows about her condition.
- You may have voiced some concern before that she has a 'serious cause' for her symptoms.
- The scenario implies that she has caecal carcinoma (although diverticular disease is a possibility).
- Remember that she is an independent and rather stoical lady who had to be persuaded to come to the Emergency Department by a worried neighbour.
- Prepare a diagram of the colon, showing the site of the lesion and illustrating the planned surgical procedure.
- The positive aspect of the scenario is that there is no evidence of intra-abdominal metastasis on the ultrasound.

Approach

Medical

- Ask her if she knows why she had the barium enema and apologise for the discomfort it caused.
- Explain that you have the result of the barium enema, which shows that there is a lump in the right side of her bowel.
- The lump has bled and this is what has led to her needing a blood transfusion.
- Tell her that the lump is likely to be cancer – make sure that you use the word 'cancer' and avoid the words 'lesion' or 'growth'.

- Make sure that she understands the diagnosis.
- Explain that the Consultant is planning to remove the cancer tomorrow and give her an outline of what the operation (a right hemicolectomy) will involve – using the diagram you have prepared or drawing it out for her when required.
- Explain the significance of the normal scan – that there is a good chance of a full recovery.

Social

- She lives alone and may need extensive social input after discharge.
- She has a supportive neighbour who you may wish to involve at this point as there is no relative living locally, but you could offer to speak to her daughter on the telephone if she wishes.
- She may require a longer inpatient stay if there is no one to live with her at home.

Psychological

- The patient has been bereaved fairly recently and lives alone – this scenario therefore represents a further piece of bad news.
- The patient's reluctance to come into hospital may in fact represent a fear of the possible diagnosis.

Minimum requirements

- You must tell her that she has cancer.
- You must tell her that she needs an operation.
- You must reassure her that there is a good chance that she will make a complete recovery.

3   OBTAINING INFORMED CONSENT

Scenario

You are a Senior House Officer in General Surgery, working in the Outpatients Department.

Michael Smith, a 25-year-old construction worker, presents to the Outpatients Department with a painless lump in his left groin, which he has had for 3 months. He has no medical problems, but he has smoked 20 cigarettes a day for the last 10 years. He drinks 20 units of alcohol per week. He lives with his wife and two children, a 6-year-old and a 4-year-old, who he drives to school every day.

You have examined Mr Smith and found that he has a large left inguinoscrotal hernia. Systemic examination is otherwise unremarkable.

Obtain informed consent from this patient for a hernia repair.

Preparation – things to consider

- You have never met this patient before.
- He may not understand what a hernia is or that it will require surgery.
- Prepare a diagram illustrating how a hernia forms and the principles of repair.
- The scenario is pushing you towards discussing his anaesthetic risk factors (smoking) and postoperative rehabilitation (driving, lifting, etc).

Approach

Medical

- Use your diagram to explain that the lump is a hernia.
- Explain the risks of leaving the hernia alone, eg obstruction, strangulation.
- Explain that you would advise him to have an operation and describe the principles of the operative procedure, including that this may involve the use of a mesh.
- Mention the specific complications and also the more general risks of surgery and ask about previous anaesthetics.
- Any complication with an incidence of greater than 1% must be mentioned.
- Some specific complications to consider are:
  - **early complications** – haematoma and scrotal bruising, infection (where a mesh has been used this is particularly important to treat vigorously)
  - **late complications** – testicular atrophy (due to damage to the vas deferens, testicular artery or

pampiniform plexus), recurrence of the hernia (should be <2% at 5 years), an area of numbness over the base of the penis due to injury to the ilio-inguinal nerve.

- In this context, it is essential to mention the risk of damage to the testis.
- Ensure that he signs a consent form after you have answered all his questions.

Social

- This should be aimed at reducing his perioperative risk and chance of recurrence:
  - **lifting** – clarify his exact role as a 'construction worker'; explain the increased risk of recurrence if he is lifting heavy objects
  - **driving** – tell him that he can only drive when he is able to make an emergency stop without regard for his operation (ie without guarding against pain/discomfort)
  - **smoking** – discuss his smoking and associated anaesthetic risk; explain the benefits of reducing or even quitting his habit and offer help as appropriate.
- Offer to repeat your advice in the presence of his wife if he wishes, and give him a leaflet or other written information prior to coming into hospital.
- Ask if he has any questions about the surgery before you finish.

Psychological

- Depending on the exertion involved in his work, he may need to take 6 weeks off following surgery – this may affect his ability to support his family.

Minimum requirements

- You have to explain what an inguinal hernia is.
- You have to explain that he needs an operation.
- You have to explain the nature of the operation and its associated risks.
- The social issues around his family, lifestyle and work must be considered.
- Obtain informed consent.

4 EXPLAINING THE NATURE OF A SURGICAL PROCEDURE

Scenario

You are a Senior House Officer on the Vascular Surgical Unit.

The patient is a 68-year-old retired policeman who lives with his wife in a bungalow and is a keen fly-fisherman.

He has recently been admitted with an acutely ischaemic right lower limb. He smokes 20 cigarettes a day and has untreated hypertension. An angiogram revealed an occluded superficial femoral artery on the right, with reasonable collaterals but no distal run-off, and no vessels can be seen at the ankle. An electrocardiogram, echocardiogram and carotid duplex scan were all within normal limits. He underwent an embolectomy 7 days ago (at which you assisted) but his leg is no better, there is frank gangrene of his medial three toes and he is unable to move the right ankle.

You have to explain to him that he needs a below-knee amputation.

Preparation – things to consider

- You have met the patient before and therefore you should establish early on what he already understands about his leg and what he has had done.
- This scenario here is about loss of function – the issue is that he has used his retirement to concentrate on fly-fishing and you are about to tell him that he needs an amputation.
- He may already suspect the worst – he has been lying in bed with a fixed ankle and black toes for 2 days.
- He should have been told about the risk of amputation before the embolectomy.
- Prepare a diagram of the vascular system of the leg to illustrate the blockage.

Approach

Medical

- You must be absolutely clear in your own mind about the necessity for amputation here:
  - His foot is non-viable and he has a fixed ankle joint, indicating irreversible loss of function.
  - He cannot have a femoro-popliteal bypass operation as there is no distal vascular run-off.
  - In fact, the previous embolectomy was a final attempt as there was no evidence of proximal thrombus (ECG and echocardiography normal).

- Use your diagram to explain what has happened to his leg.
- You must be able to explain how to perform a below-knee amputation and the reasons why this is a much better option for him than an above-knee amputation.
- You must be prepared to offer information on the many ways in which his life afterwards can be normalised.
- You must be able to list the complications of below-knee amputation if he asks.

Social

- He lives in a bungalow and stairs are not going to be a problem. However, he is going to need a wheelchair at home and the doors may be too narrow – an occupational therapy assessment would be appropriate here.
- Arrangements can be made for any changes to his house to be made before he goes home.
- He does have someone at home with him and you should ask if he would like you to contact his wife in order to have a joint discussion.

Psychological

- Empathy is the key to the success of your approach in this scenario and you should try to understand the psychological consequences of losing his leg for this active man.
- The use of a prosthetic limb will be crucial to his rehabilitation and this should be mentioned.
- He will be able to drive a car and walk to the river to fish but he may need assistance.

Minimum requirements

- You must explain that he needs an amputation, as all other possible treatments have been explored.
- You must empathise with how this operation will change his lifestyle.
- You must offer to help him with rehabilitation and explain how this will be achieved.

5   OBTAINING CONSENT FOR ORGAN DONATION

Scenario

You are a Senior House Officer in General Surgery.

A 22-year-old man was admitted with a head injury following a motorbike accident 2 days ago. He was not wearing a helmet. He was unconscious on arrival and never regained consciousness. A CT scan of his brain on admission revealed several large extradural and subdural haematomas which were not amenable to surgical drainage.

His mother, father and two brothers have maintained a round-the-clock vigil in ITU, where he has remained intubated, ventilated and paralysed. A CT scan repeated yesterday showed considerable deterioration in the brain insult.

He has been examined by two senior anaesthetists and has been pronounced brainstem-dead.

You have been asked to discuss, and obtain consent for, organ donation from the father. This patient did not have a donor card in his wallet.

Preparation – things to consider

- You are likely to have met the father previously over the last 2 days.
- The scenario suggests the family are close (they have kept a vigil by his bed).
- The family is likely to have noticed the lack of improvement.
- They have probably been given a good deal of clinical information already, but they may not understand that there is no expectation of improvement.
- You are asked to discuss organ donation and it is very important that you move on to this relatively quickly – a common pitfall is to spend too much time here empathising with the grieving relatives, although empathy is essential.
- In this case, the patient was not carrying a donor card. The law states that relatives must be in agreement, whether or not the patient carries a donor card.
- The way to begin this scenario, as in any situation when you have met the interviewee before, is to ask what they already know.

Approach

Re-introduce yourself only if the actor implies he does not remember you.

Explaining 'brain death'

- Establish the starting point by asking the father what he knows about the current state of his son's injuries.
- Explain the seriousness of the head injury, which has led to bleeding and extensive brain damage.
- Explain that the extent of this damage means that his son can no longer breathe for himself and that he is therefore on a ventilator.
- Ask at this point whether he understands the significance of what you are saying.
- Ask him if he understands what 'brain-dead' means and emphasise that it is impossible for his son to regain consciousness.
- Pause and allow him to take this in; be prepared to react if the actor begins to cry – offer tissues if available and decide in advance whether you feel comfortable holding the actor's hand (be led by the actor's reactions).
- Say, 'I'm sorry' and wait before moving on.

Organ donation

- Approach the organ donation subject carefully.
- Be direct – we would anticipate that the father has some understanding that organ donation is an important part of the care of the critically ill.
- Perhaps begin with, 'There's something else I need to talk to you about . . .' and explain that although his son's brain is dead, blood is flowing to all the other organs and that the artificial ventilator is breathing for him.
- Mention the benefit to others of organ transplantation.
- Ask if his son had ever indicated a wish for his organs to be donated.
- Be prepared to give a list of the organs that may be used (liver, heart, lungs, corneas, kidneys) and to discuss the specific details of the process that would take place, including the use of a regional transplant coordinator.
- Reiterate that there is no chance of improvement and that time is of the essence in order to avoid any irreparable damage to the organs.

Do not force a discussion if the father insists he will not even consider organ donation as an option, or pressure him into making a decision.

Conclude by telling him that you will return to discuss things when he has had a chance to think some more about the situation and to discuss it with his family ('I know this is a lot to absorb . . .').

Invite him to go back and see his son now if he wants to.

Minimum requirements

- You must tell the father that his son is brain-dead and that he will not regain consciousness.
- You must show empathy and compassion.
- You must discuss, and preferably obtain consent for, organ donation.
- You should allow him to be with his son again at the end.

6   EXPLAINING HOSPITAL CARE

Scenario

You are a Senior House Officer in Trauma and Ortho-paedics.

Last week, you admitted a 90-year-old lady with dementia who lives in a nursing home. She had tripped over when being helped to the bathroom. As a result of this fall, she sustained a right fractured neck of femur. She was admitted to hospital and was found to be severely dehydrated. Surgery was delayed for 2 days while she was being resuscitated.

The patient's daughter lives in South Wales and she was con-tacted before her mother was taken to the operating theatre for a hemiarthroplasty. Consent for the operation was given by two registered practitioners, as per local protocol. After the operation, she developed atrial fibrillation and this was treated with amiodarone. Now she has developed a right lower lobe pneumonia.

Her daughter arrived yesterday and has been very distressed by what has happened to her mother – she has made an appointment to see you after you have finished your morning in the Outpatients Department and is waiting in the office on the Orthopaedic Ward.

Preparation – things to consider

- You have not met this relative before and she is likely to be more confused than angry about what has happened to her mother.
- Clearly this situation is very common in clinical practice but nevertheless it is very distressing for relatives when complications occur as a result of surgery.
- Questions in her mind might include:
  - Why was surgery not performed immediately?
  - Were any other treatment options (other than surgery) possible?
  - Why has she suffered these two separate postoperative complications?
  - Is the hospital (and the orthopaedic team in particular) incompetent?
- She will be looking for thorough and detailed explanations, with a promise that you will keep her personally informed of developments from now on.
- Prepare a diagram of the hip showing the fracture and the prosthesis used to fix the fracture.

Approach

Medical

- Most of this session is likely to be taken up with explaining what has happened and reassurance that this lady's mother is being cared for properly at the hospital.
- Introduce yourself as one of the team that has been caring for her mother.
- From the start, you should take on some personal responsibility for the patient's problems.
- Use your diagram to illustrate the injury that she had, distancing yourself and the hospital from any involvement in this.
- Allow her to ask some questions and explain the reason for the delay before surgery, mentioning that she arrived in the hospital dehydrated.
- Take some time to emphasise that a fractured neck of femur indicates a poor prognosis because of co-morbidity.
- Discuss the specific reasons (anaesthetic, atelectasis, risk of infection) that contributed to the postoperative problems, giving an indication of how common these are, and answer her questions honestly. Paint a realistic picture of how serious things are.

Social

- The family may be concerned about the safety of the nursing home, as she fell there.
- Be sympathetic about this but remember that **this is not your responsibility**.
- If further help is required regarding future residential placement, explain that you will ensure social services are involved.

Psychological

- Dealing with elderly relatives with dementia is a problem for many families but it is often only when additional problems occur that tensions between family members become apparent.
- Your role is to be sympathetic and to explain the medical aspects of the case as clearly as possible without attributing any blame to any individual.
- You should not make any guarantees about when she will be discharged.

- If she asks whether there is any chance her mother will die, you must be honest.

Minimum requirements
- You must discuss the medical problems honestly and appropriately.
- The relative should leave you feeling reassured that her mother is being cared for properly.

7   ENROLMENT INTO CLINICAL TRIALS

Scenario

You are an Orthopaedic Registrar in the Outpatients Department. A 64-year-old lady is scheduled to undergo a right total hip replacement for osteoarthritis in 3 weeks' time.

Your department is involved in recruiting patients into a clinical trial for a multinational pharmaceutical company. A prospective, randomised, double-blind clinical trial has been designed to compare a new subcutaneous anticoagulant (MX00432Y) with low molecular weight heparin for thromboprophylaxis in patients who are undergoing total hip replacement. The only contraindication to participation in the trial is any history of bleeding disorder.

Your Senior House Officer has already obtained her consent for the surgical procedure itself, but you have to obtain informed consent from this lady in order to enrol her into the trial.

Preparation – things to consider

- You have never met this lady before.
- You may have to go over the details of the surgery again.
- She may well not have been told previously that she will have daily low molecular weight heparin, or even that there is a risk of deep vein thrombosis associated with this procedure.
- This lady may have preconceptions about clinical trials, and may need to have some of the background to the trial explained in detail.

Approach

Medical

- The first objective is clarification that this lady understands the operation.
- Ask the lady to explain the operation to you, as she understands it. This not only reinforces her knowledge of what is about to happen to her, but it also gives you time to think about what you are gong to say next.
- Explain the reasons for administering perioperative anticoagulants and the hospital's protocol. (Note that the risk of postoperative deep vein thrombosis in a patient who is not receiving thromboprophylaxis during a total hip replacement can be 20%–40%.)
- Contraindications to therapy should be actively sought, such as a history of bleeding disorders.
- Do not dwell on any other medical problems that are not relevant to this situation, as this only wastes time.

Social

- There is not much to deal with in this respect in this case as the social issues would have been dealt with in the preoperative work-up.

Psychological

- She may be anxious as she has been recalled to Outpatients ahead of her date for surgery; she may even have been told that the appointment is to discuss 'research'.
- You must allay any fears that she may have of being used as a 'guinea pig' in a medical experiment.
- Explain in layman's terms exactly what a prospective, randomised, double-blind clinical trial is.
- Describe any risks and benefits of being involved in the trial, such as the risk of allergic reaction and the potential to improve her current condition.
- Make it absolutely clear that there will be no disadvantages if she declines to take part in the trial.
- She has to either sign the consent form or decline to take part, but give her ample opportunity to think about the information or offer to see her again if necessary, perhaps with her partner.

Minimum requirements

- You have to explain why anticoagulation is required.
- You have to explain the potential risks of anticoagulation.
- You have to explain clearly what taking part in the trial will involve.
- You have to reassure the patient that this trial is ethical and that it is hoped that it will contribute significantly to the body of knowledge in this medical field.

8   EXPLAINING THE SIGNIFICANCE OF A DIAGNOSIS

Scenario

You are a Senior House Officer in the Vascular Surgery Out-patients Clinic.

A 65-year-old retired bus driver was referred by his GP to a urologist to investigate his poor urinary stream, hesitancy and nocturia. As part of the work-up, the urologist organised an ultrasound scan of the abdomen. The ultrasound report includes the following sentence: 'There is a 6.4-cm abdominal aortic aneurysm.'

His wife recently died of a stroke, 2 weeks before their fortieth wedding anniversary. His son lives abroad and there is no other social support. He walks half a mile to the shops every day to bet on the horses and takes no regular medication.

The urologist has made a diagnosis of benign prostatic hyperplasia and has referred the patient to your Consultant.

You have to explain to this patient how you are going to manage him and discuss the implications of his vascular diagnosis.

Preparation – things to consider

- You have never met this man before.
- He has no idea what is wrong with him other than his urological symptoms.
- You will be required to explain what an abdominal aortic aneurysm is (this would be facilitated by a diagram) and what the significance of this diagnosis is, mentioning the risks of rupture and embolus in lay terms.
- Do not wander into a discussion about the urological problems – this would be non-productive in terms of the instruction given.

Approach

Medical

- He has an abdominal aortic aneurysm that requires elective repair.
- The risk of rupture of aneurysms of this size is 10%–15% per annum.
- The operative mortality is 5% (less in specialist centres) but the mortality following rupture would be 50%.
- He would be considered a suitable candidate for surgery, especially as his health is otherwise good.

Social

- He lives alone and has no social support nearby.
- Postoperatively, this will be an issue in terms of his recovery and he may need to have a period of convalescence, for example in a GP hospital bed.
- His son is a long way away but you would gain extra marks for offering to speak to the son on a separate occasion.
- If the nearest shops are half a mile away, he will need help at home when he is discharged, eg home help, meals on wheels.

Psychological

- This patient is likely to be depressed, given the information in the scenario.
- Do not ask the patient about this directly – but if he brings it up, you should consider how this might be dealt with within the limitations of a busy vascular clinic.

Minimum requirements

- You have to tell the patient that he has an abdominal aortic aneurysm and what this is.
- You have to tell him that he requires surgery.
- You have to tell him that there is a risk of his dying, with or without the operation.

9 REASSURING A PATIENT WITH NEGATIVE TEST RESULTS

Scenario

You are a Senior House Officer in the Department of Urology.

A 46-year-old City company director has been seen in the Urological Outpatient Clinic for the investigation of haematuria. He has no other medical problems but smokes heavily and drinks 30 units of alcohol a week. Initially, his GP treated him with a week of antibiotics. Clinical examination was normal and he has now had mid-stream specimen of urine and prostate-specific antigen tests, an ultrasound scan of the renal tract and a flexible cystoscopy, none of which have shown any abnormality.

The patient has returned to Outpatients to discuss the results of his tests and he is very anxious as no apparent cause of the haematuria has been uncovered.

Preparation – things to consider

- This session will be one of reassurance.
- It often happens that you will be provided with much more information than this, and the temptation is to try and think of some other test that **could** be performed.
- The point is that sometimes there is nothing seriously wrong and the goal in this situation is simply to communicate this to a patient, so that they can be reassured.
- It may help to prepare a diagram of the lower urinary tract which illustrates all the various places where haematuria could have originated.

Approach

Medical

- Introduce yourself and ask him what he understands has happened to him so far.
- He may have already gathered a great deal of information from the Consultant in the clinic.
- It is possible that he has done some background research (reading or surfing the Internet) to find out more.
- Do not patronise him by taking the discussion to too simple a level (the scenario tells you he is a company director), but avoid confusing him with medical jargon.
- Tell him what the serious causes of haematuria are and what steps have been taken to exclude these in a systematic manner.
- Explain that although nothing is a certainty in medicine, nothing is likely to be seriously wrong here.

- The most likely cause of his symptoms was a urinary tract infection, which was adequately treated by his GP.
- He may bring up the possibility of sexually transmitted risk factors for his symptoms, which you could discuss, but avoid initiating a discussion around this.

Social and psychological

- Many patients need an answer to everything and some expect the worst when in fact there may be a very straightforward explanation for their symptoms.
- This man is a company director, which may mean that he is under a great deal of stress – haematuria is likely to be an unwelcome extra worry.
- You could take the opportunity to discuss lifestyle risks with him – quitting smoking, moderate alcohol intake and stress management.

Minimum requirements

- You must reassure him adequately that nothing serious is wrong.
- You must identify any specific fears and discuss these openly.
- Be prepared to discuss any further issues that he introduces honestly.

10 'I'M ONLY SEEING THE CONSULTANT'

Scenario

You are the Senior House Officer in the Breast Clinic and the Consultant is unwell today, so has not come along to Out-patients.

A 53-year-old physiotherapist has been referred by her GP with a suspicious lump in the right breast. Her sister has recently died of advanced breast cancer. Previously healthy, the patient is nulliparous and has been taking the oral contraceptive pill for several years. She has been researching on the Internet and found out that both these factors contribute to a higher risk of breast cancer.

The Breast Care Nurse has already seen this patient and has commented to you that she is 'insisting on only seeing the consultant'. The problem is that the patient was very nervous about coming to the clinic and her husband is adamant that he does not want her to leave without the appropriate investigations, which the Breast Care Nurse cannot order.

Leaving out the clinical examination, assess this patient's risk and order whichever tests you think are indicated.

Preparation – things to consider

Consider the reasons why the patient only wants to see the Consultant:

- She is a physiotherapist and wants the 'best available' opinion.
- She is very anxious about the probable diagnosis.
- Her GP may have made a comment about the particular skills of this Consultant.
- Her sister has recently died and there may be some areas of concern in the patient's management.

Approach

Concentrate on being completely professional and demonstrating to this patient that, despite her reservations, you are capable of doing your job.

Medical

- This lady clearly has a high risk of breast cancer and now presents with a lump in the breast.
- Take a full history of the lump, thoroughly explore the risk factors for breast cancer, and assess her risk for surgery.
- The investigations required would be a mammogram and a fine-needle aspiration of the lump.

- You may want to proceed to chromosomal analysis for *BRCA1* and *BRCA2* genes.
- Make arrangements for follow-up, perhaps at next week's Breast Clinic, when the consultant may be present.

Social

- She is married but has not had children (although she may have adopted).
- Her husband is clearly very worried about her but you are not given any other information about the home situation.
- She works as a physiotherapist and may be worried about the work or financial implications of having investigations and possibly surgery.

Psychological

- You may want to address the psychological issues first in this scenario.
- You should acknowledge that this lady would prefer to see the Consultant, and show that you respect this choice.
- Apologise for the Consultant's not being available and explain why he is absent.
- Tell the patient that you will discuss her case with him on his return and perhaps offer to ask the Consultant to telephone her over the next few days or to arrange to see her with all the results.
- Explain that the team's role today is not to make a decision about treatment but simply to ensure that the appropriate investigations are organised.
- If she still believes that you are not the right person to see her, then it is reasonable to offer to rebook her for the next clinic when the Consultant is back.

Minimum requirements

- You must offer an explanation for why the Consultant is absent.
- You must formulate a plan for the appropriate management of this lady in light of her probable diagnosis.
- You must act appropriately in order to allay the patient's concerns that you are not the right person to organise the investigations.

INDEX

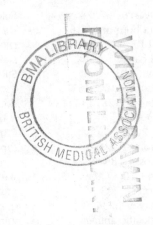